Medical Coder

-

The Comprehensive Guide

by

VIRUTI SHIVAN

Masters in Clinical Psychology (Major)

"In books, as in life, it's not the size or looks but the content that matters."

Introduction

Welcome to the exciting world of medical coding, a crucial component of the healthcare industry that bridges the gap between health care providers and the billing offices. "Medical Coder - The Comprehensive Guide" is your passport to understanding and mastering this complex, yet fascinating field. This book is designed to offer you a deep dive into the realm of medical coding, providing you with the knowledge and tools necessary to embark on a rewarding career.

Why Medical Coding?

At first glance, medical coding might seem like a series of incomprehensible symbols and numbers. However, these codes are the backbone of the healthcare billing process, ensuring that health care providers are reimbursed for the services they provide. But medical coding is more than just about numbers; it's a dynamic field that requires a keen understanding of medical terminology, anatomy, coding systems, and the laws that govern healthcare.

A Guide for All

Whether you are a complete novice curious about the field, a student embarking on your studies, or a seasoned professional looking to brush up on the latest in coding standards, this guide is tailored for you. With detailed chapters on ICD-10, CPT, and

HCPCS coding, as well as insights into billing, compliance, and the technology that's shaping the future of coding, this book covers every angle.

Practical and Engaging

Our approach is both practical and engaging, blending theoretical knowledge with real-world applications. We understand that learning medical coding can be daunting, so we've sprinkled the content with practical examples, fun facts, and exercises to test your understanding and keep you engaged. Remember, this is a field where continuous learning is part of the job description, and our goal is to make that learning as enjoyable and effective as possible.

Ethics and Compliance

The importance of ethics and compliance cannot be overstated in medical coding. This guide emphasizes the ethical considerations in coding and the significance of accurate, honest coding practices. You'll learn about the regulations that govern healthcare and how to navigate the complex compliance landscape.

Your Journey Begins Here

As you turn the pages of this guide, you'll embark on a journey through the intricacies of medical coding. Each chapter is designed to build on the previous one, gradually expanding your knowledge and skills. By the end of this book, you'll have a solid foundation in medical coding, ready to tackle the challenges of the field with confidence and expertise.

Let's embark on this journey together, unraveling the mysteries of medical coding and unlocking the doors to a fulfilling career. Welcome to "Medical Coder - The Comprehensive Guide."

Chapter 1: Introduction to Medical Coding

1.1. The Role of a Medical Coder

Imagine you're a detective, but instead of solving crimes, you're deciphering the story of a patient's journey through the healthcare system. This is the role of a medical coder: a crucial player in healthcare, whose job is to translate every diagnosis, procedure, and medical service into standardized codes. But why, you might ask, is this translation so important?

The Heart of Healthcare Billing

At its core, medical coding is the transformation of healthcare diagnosis, procedures, treatments, and equipment into universal medical alphanumeric codes. These codes come from medical records such as the doctor's notes, laboratory results, and radiologic findings. Medical coders ensure that these records are accurately represented in the billing process, facilitating a smooth transaction between healthcare providers and insurers.

Beyond the Codes

Medical coding is not just about assigning codes; it's a complex process that involves understanding the patient's story, the healthcare provider's actions, and the nuances of medical terminology. Coders must be adept at reading and interpreting medical records, but they also need a solid grasp of the coding guidelines for the ICD-10-CM (International Classification of Diseases, Tenth Revision, Clinical Modification), CPT (Current Procedural Terminology), and HCPCS (Healthcare Common Procedure Coding System).

The Impact of Accurate Coding

Accurate coding is vital for several reasons:

- **Reimbursement:** It ensures that healthcare providers are paid correctly and promptly for the services they deliver.

- **Compliance:** It helps in adhering to the coding standards set by laws and regulations, thereby avoiding legal issues.

- **Quality Care:** It supports the evaluation of healthcare services and outcomes, facilitating improvements in patient care.

A Career of Lifelong Learning

One of the most exciting aspects of being a medical coder is the opportunity for continuous learning. Medical science is always advancing, and with it, coding guidelines and regulations are regularly updated. This dynamic environment requires coders to stay informed and adaptable, making it a perfect career for those who love to learn and solve puzzles.

A Day in the Life

So, what does a day in the life of a medical coder look like? It involves a lot of detective work: sifting through patient records, consulting coding manuals, and using coding software. Coders work closely with healthcare providers to clarify any ambiguities in the records and ensure that every piece of the patient's story is accurately coded.

Medical coders are the unsung heroes of the healthcare world, playing a key role in ensuring the financial and operational efficiency of healthcare services. Their work may be behind the scenes, but it's absolutely vital to the healthcare industry's success.

As we delve deeper into the world of medical coding in the following chapters, keep in mind the critical role of medical coders. They're not just translators of medical jargon into codes; they're essential contributors to the overall healthcare delivery system, ensuring accuracy, compliance, and the facilitation of quality care.

1.2. Overview of Healthcare Systems

Before we dive deeper into the specifics of medical coding, let's zoom out and take a bird's-eye view of the healthcare systems within which medical coders operate. Understanding the broader context helps illuminate why coding is so integral to the function and efficiency of healthcare delivery.

The Complex Ecosystem of Healthcare

Healthcare systems can be visualized as intricate ecosystems comprising various entities: hospitals, clinics, private practices, insurance companies, government programs, and patients themselves. Each plays a pivotal role in the health and well-being of the population, and at the center of this complex web is the exchange of information and financial transactions enabled by medical coding.

Types of Healthcare Systems

Globally, healthcare systems take on different forms, influenced by economic, political, and social factors. However, they generally fall into a few categories:

- **Single-Payer Systems:** In these systems, a single public agency manages health care financing, and the delivery of care remains largely in private hands. The Canadian healthcare system is a prime example.

- **National Health Insurance Models:** These systems also rely on taxpayer-funded insurance for every citizen, but the care providers are private. South Korea's healthcare system exemplifies this model.

- **Private Insurance Systems:** The United States is unique in its reliance on a predominantly private insurance system, supplemented by public insurance programs like Medicare and Medicaid for specific population segments.

- **Out-of-Pocket Models:** In many parts of the world, healthcare services are paid for by the patient out of pocket, which can lead to disparities in access to care.

The Role of Coding in Healthcare Systems

No matter the system, medical coding is the universal language that allows for the efficient processing of healthcare data. This includes:

- **Billing and Reimbursement:** Coding translates services into billable codes, ensuring providers are reimbursed.

- **Healthcare Analysis:** Codes are used to track health trends, manage population health, and guide public health policy.

- **Insurance Processing:** Codes help insurers determine coverage and process claims efficiently.

Challenges and Opportunities

Each healthcare system presents unique challenges and opportunities for medical coders. For instance, in a system with multiple private insurers, coders must navigate a complex landscape of coverage plans and coding requirements. Conversely, in single-payer systems, while there may be more uniformity in coding practices, the volume and complexity of services coded can be immense.

Adapting to Change

Healthcare is an ever-evolving field, impacted by technological advancements, policy changes, and societal needs. Medical coders are at the forefront of adapting to these changes, ensuring that the language of coding meets the demands of modern healthcare delivery. This adaptability not only ensures the sustainability of healthcare systems but also highlights the critical role coders play in the health of populations.

A Foundation for Future Learning

As we delve into the specifics of medical coding in subsequent chapters, keep this overview in mind. The context in which coders work is as important as the codes themselves, influencing how they approach their tasks and the strategies they use to ensure accuracy and compliance. The ecosystem of healthcare is complex, but at its heart, it seeks to deliver quality care to all—and medical coders are key players in making that a reality.

1.3. Ethics and Compliance in Medical Coding

In the realm of medical coding, where the translation of healthcare services into a standardized language intersects with billing and insurance claims, ethics and compliance are not just buzzwords—they are foundational pillars. The integrity of medical coders directly impacts the financial and operational aspects of healthcare providers and the trust of patients in the healthcare system. Let's explore why ethics and compliance hold such paramount importance in medical coding and how they influence the profession.

The Ethical Framework

At its core, ethics in medical coding is about doing the right thing, even when no one is watching. This includes:

- **Accuracy:** Ensuring that codes accurately reflect the patient's diagnosis and the services rendered.

- **Confidentiality:** Protecting patient information with the utmost care and in accordance with laws like HIPAA (Health Insurance Portability and Accountability Act).

- **Integrity:** Avoiding the temptation to manipulate codes for higher reimbursement or to meet productivity benchmarks dishonestly.

Ethical challenges can arise in scenarios where there is pressure to upcode (report more severe diagnoses or procedures than were actually performed) or downcode (report less severe diagnoses or procedures to avoid scrutiny). Coders must navigate these pressures by adhering to ethical principles, ensuring that their work accurately reflects the care provided.

Compliance: The Rulebook for Coders

Compliance in medical coding refers to following laws, regulations, and guidelines that govern the practice. This includes:

- **Federal and State Regulations:** Adhering to healthcare laws, including those related to billing and privacy.

- **Coding Guidelines:** Following the specific rules set forth by coding systems like ICD-10, CPT, and HCPCS.

- **Payer Policies:** Understanding and complying with the individual policies of Medicare, Medicaid, and private insurance companies.

Compliance is not static; it requires ongoing education and awareness as laws and guidelines evolve. Medical coders play a critical role in preventing fraud and abuse by ensuring that their coding practices meet legal and ethical standards.

Why It Matters

The consequences of unethical or non-compliant coding can be severe, impacting not just the coder but the healthcare provider, the payer, and ultimately, the patient. Penalties can include fines, legal action, and damage to reputation. On a larger scale, unethical coding practices can contribute to the rising costs of healthcare and erode trust in the healthcare system.

Building a Culture of Integrity

Creating a culture of integrity within the medical coding profession involves:

- **Education:** Ongoing training in ethical practices and compliance for all coders.

- **Resources:** Providing coders with the tools and support they need to make ethical decisions.

- **Open Communication:** Encouraging a work environment where coders feel comfortable raising ethical concerns.

The Human Element

Remember, behind every code is a patient with a story. Ethical and compliant coding practices ensure that this story is told accurately, respecting the patient's journey through the healthcare system. It's about more than just getting the codes right; it's about upholding the trust patients place in healthcare providers and the broader system.

As we delve into the nuts and bolts of medical coding in the chapters that follow, keep the principles of ethics and compliance at the forefront. They are not just guidelines but commitments to excellence, integrity, and the well-being of patients in the healthcare system.

1.4. Career Opportunities in Medical Coding

Embarking on a career in medical coding opens a world of possibilities. Far from being a monotonous task of translating healthcare services into codes, the field of medical coding offers a variety of pathways, each with its unique challenges and rewards. Let's explore the landscape of career opportunities in medical coding, highlighting the diverse roles that await those ready to dive into this essential sector of the healthcare industry.

The Core of Medical Coding Careers

At its heart, a career in medical coding involves working with healthcare providers, billing offices, and insurance companies to ensure accurate and efficient processing of medical claims. But within this core function lies a spectrum of roles:

- **Inpatient and Outpatient Coders:** These professionals specialize in coding for services rendered in hospitals (inpatient) and ambulatory settings (outpatient). Each setting requires a deep understanding of specific coding guidelines and patient types.

- **Specialty Coders:** Focusing on areas like cardiology, orthopedics, pediatrics, or oncology, specialty coders possess detailed knowledge of the procedures and services commonly encountered in their chosen fields.

- **Auditing and Compliance:** Coders with experience and additional certifications may move into roles that audit coding for accuracy and compliance, ensuring that coding practices meet all legal and regulatory requirements.

- **Education and Training:** Experienced coders can also transition into roles as educators, teaching aspiring coders in academic settings or providing ongoing education for healthcare providers on coding standards and best practices.

**Expanding Horizons

The field of medical coding is evolving, and with it, new career opportunities are emerging:

- **Remote Coding:** Advances in technology and the digitalization of medical records have made remote coding a viable and increasingly popular option. This allows for greater flexibility and the opportunity to work for organizations across the country or even globally.

- **Consulting:** Experienced coders may offer their expertise as consultants, helping practices optimize their coding processes, navigate compliance issues, or transition to new coding standards.

- **Health Information Management (HIM):** Coders with an interest in the broader aspects of medical records and patient information might pursue careers in HIM, focusing on managing and safeguarding patient data.

Skills That Open Doors

Success in medical coding requires a blend of hard and soft skills:

- **Analytical Skills:** The ability to interpret and apply complex coding guidelines is fundamental.

- **Attention to Detail:** Precision is crucial, as small coding errors can have significant implications.

- **Communication:** Coders must effectively communicate with healthcare providers to clarify documentation and with billing staff to resolve coding queries.

- **Adaptability:** The healthcare landscape is always changing, and coders must stay current with new coding standards and technologies.

Certification: Your Key to Advancement

Certification through recognized organizations like the AAPC (American Academy of Professional Coders) or AHIMA (American Health Information Management Association) is often a requirement for employment and a stepping stone to advanced career opportunities. Certifications such as the Certified Professional Coder (CPC) and Certified Coding Specialist (CCS) are highly regarded in the industry.

A Future Bright with Possibility

The demand for skilled medical coders is expected to grow, driven by the expansion of healthcare services and the increasing complexity of medical billing and insurance claims. With a foundation in medical coding, you can build a career that is not only financially rewarding but also contributes to the efficient and ethical delivery of healthcare services.

Embarking on a career in medical coding means joining a community of professionals dedicated to excellence, integrity, and the continuous pursuit of knowledge. Whether you're drawn to the analytical challenge of coding, the satisfaction of supporting patient care, or the opportunities for advancement and specialization, medical coding offers a fulfilling and dynamic career path.

1.5. Exercise: 10 MCQs with Answers at the End

Test your understanding of the fundamentals of medical coding with these multiple-choice questions. Covering topics from the role of medical coders to career opportunities, these questions are designed to reinforce your learning from the first chapter. Answers are provided at the end for you to check your work.

Questions

1. What is the primary role of a medical coder?

   A. Diagnosing patient illnesses

   B. Translating healthcare services into standardized codes

   C. Directly billing patients for healthcare services

   D. Providing medical advice based on patient records

2. Which coding system is used for diagnosing diseases and conditions?

   A. CPT

   B. ICD-10-CM

C. HCPCS

D. E/M

3. What does HIPAA stand for?

   A. Health Insurance Portability and Accountability Act

   B. Healthcare Information and Privacy Assurance Act

   C. Health Insurance Protection and Privacy Act

   D. Healthcare Informatics and Patient Assistance Act

4. In which setting would an outpatient coder most likely work?

   A. Hospital inpatient departments

   B. Ambulatory surgical centers

   C. Long-term care facilities

   D. Home health agencies

5. What is the main reason for the ethical coding of medical records?

   A. To ensure the coder's job security

   B. To maximize the healthcare provider's revenue

   C. To ensure accurate and fair billing practices

   D. To simplify the coder's workload

6. Which of the following is a certification for medical coders?

A. Registered Health Information Technician (RHIT)

B. Certified Professional Coder (CPC)

C. Licensed Practical Nurse (LPN)

D. Certified Medical Assistant (CMA)

7. The process of checking coding accuracy and compliance is known as:

A. Auditing

B. Billing

C. Transcription

D. Documentation

8. What skill is crucial for medical coders to accurately assign codes?

A. Negotiation

B. Mathematical calculation

C. Attention to detail

D. Physical stamina

9. Which career path involves teaching new coders and providing ongoing education?

A. Medical billing specialist

B. Coding auditor

C. Health information manager

D. Coding educator

10. Remote coding has become more viable due to:

    A. The preference for paper-based records

    B. Advances in telehealth services

    C. The digitalization of medical records

    D. Increased patient demand for in-person consultations

Answers

1. B. Translating healthcare services into standardized codes

2. B. ICD-10-CM

3. A. Health Insurance Portability and Accountability Act

4. B. Ambulatory surgical centers

5. C. To ensure accurate and fair billing practices

6. B. Certified Professional Coder (CPC)

7. A. Auditing

8. C. Attention to detail

9. D. Coding educator

10. C. The digitalization of medical records

Use these questions as a tool to review your knowledge and identify areas where you may need to focus more attention. Remember, practice and continuous learning are key to mastering medical coding.

Chapter 2: Medical Terminology and Anatomy

2.1. Basic Medical Terminology

Diving into the world of medical coding without a solid grasp of medical terminology is like trying to read a map without knowing the symbols. Medical terminology forms the bedrock upon which all coding is built, enabling coders to accurately translate medical reports into coded data. This section introduces you to the basics of medical terminology, breaking down the complex language of medicine into understandable parts.

The Language of Medicine

Medical terminology is a specialized language used by healthcare professionals to describe the human body, its functions, diseases, procedures, and treatments. It originates from Latin and Greek languages, giving it a universal aspect that transcends geographical boundaries. Understanding this language is crucial for medical coders, as it allows them to interpret the details of medical reports accurately.

Breaking Down the Words

Medical terms can be broken down into components that, when combined, give a precise description of a condition or procedure. These components include:

- **Root Words:** The base of the term, often indicating the part of the body or the basic idea (e.g., "cardi" refers to the heart).

- **Prefixes:** Added to the beginning of a root word to modify its meaning (e.g., "brady-" means slow, so "bradycardia" means slow heart rate).

- **Suffixes:** Added to the end of a root word to indicate a procedure, condition, disease, or part of speech (e.g., "-itis" means inflammation, so "arthritis" is inflammation of a joint).

- **Combining Forms:** A root word plus a vowel that makes the term easier to pronounce (e.g., "oste/o" refers to bone).

Common Prefixes and Suffixes

Understanding common prefixes and suffixes can help demystify many medical terms. For example:

- Prefixes like "hyper-" (excessive) and "hypo-" (under) can describe conditions like hypertension (high blood pressure) or hypoglycemia (low blood sugar).

- Suffixes such as "-ectomy" (surgical removal) and "-plasty" (surgical repair) can help identify procedures like appendectomy (removal of the appendix) or rhinoplasty (surgical repair of the nose).

Anatomy of a Medical Term

Let's take the term "electrocardiogram" as an example:

- "Electro-" (prefix) refers to electricity.

- "Cardi" (root) refers to the heart.

- "-ogram" (suffix) refers to a recording or picture.

Together, "electrocardiogram" describes a recording of the heart's electrical activity.

Practical Application

For medical coders, understanding medical terminology is not just about memorizing words; it's about understanding the story behind a patient's healthcare encounter. This knowledge enables coders to navigate through medical records with precision, ensuring accurate representation of the patient's story in the coded data.

Building Your Vocabulary

The best way to master medical terminology is through continuous learning and practice. Start with the basics, and gradually add new terms to your vocabulary. Use flashcards, join study groups, and apply what you learn in real-world coding scenarios. Remember, each term you learn not only enhances your coding skills but also deepens your understanding of the complex world of healthcare.

As you become more familiar with medical terminology, you'll find it becomes a powerful tool in your coding toolkit, enabling you to capture the nuances of patient care with accuracy and confidence. Welcome to the fascinating journey of medical language—a journey that is both challenging and incredibly rewarding.

2.2. Human Anatomy for Coders

Grasping the vast and intricate field of human anatomy is akin to learning the geography of an unknown land for medical coders. It's about understanding the landscape where medical narratives unfold—each organ, system, and structure plays a role in the patient's health story. This knowledge is not just academic; it's practical, enhancing a coder's ability to accurately translate medical records into the universal language of coding.

The Body's Systems: A Roadmap

Think of the human body as a complex, highly organized structure, divided into several systems, each with a specific function yet interconnected in maintaining health and homeostasis. Here's a brief tour:

- **Skeletal System:** The framework of bones and joints that supports the body, protects organs, and produces blood cells.

- **Muscular System:** Comprising muscles and tendons, this system facilitates movement, stability, and posture.

- **Cardiovascular System:** Includes the heart and blood vessels, pumping blood to distribute oxygen and nutrients while removing waste.

- **Respiratory System:** Consists of the lungs and airways, enabling oxygen intake and carbon dioxide expulsion.

- **Digestive System:** A complex network from the mouth to the anus, breaking down food, absorbing nutrients, and expelling waste.

- **Nervous System:** The brain, spinal cord, and nerves constitute this system, orchestrating bodily functions through electrical and chemical signals.

- **Endocrine System:** Comprised of glands that release hormones, it regulates processes like growth, metabolism, and reproduction.

- **Urinary System:** The kidneys, bladder, and associated ducts work to remove waste and regulate fluid and electrolyte balance.

- **Reproductive System:** The organs involved in reproduction, differing significantly between males and females.

- **Integumentary System:** Encompassing the skin, hair, and nails, it protects against environmental damage and regulates temperature.

- **Lymphatic and Immune System:** A network of lymph nodes, vessels, and organs that work to defend against infection and disease.

Why Anatomy Matters for Coders

Understanding anatomy elevates a coder's work from mere data entry to a critical component of healthcare delivery. It allows coders to:

- **Ensure Precision:** Differentiate between procedures performed on similar but distinct anatomical parts.

- **Anticipate Errors:** Recognize when a procedure code doesn't match the diagnosed condition based on anatomical impossibilities.

- **Facilitate Communication:** Engage more effectively with healthcare providers, querying with informed precision when documentation seems unclear or incomplete.

Anatomy in Action

Let's consider a coding scenario: A patient undergoes a laparoscopic cholecystectomy. Knowing that "laparoscopic" refers to a minimally invasive technique using small incisions, and "cholecystectomy" is the removal of the gallbladder, a coder can accurately assign the procedure code. This accuracy is crucial for billing, medical records, and even the patient's understanding of their own care.

Tools for Learning

For coders, the journey through anatomy doesn't require memorizing every detail but understanding the blueprint. Utilize anatomy atlases, online courses, and interactive tools designed for medical professionals. Engage with coding scenarios that challenge your understanding, and collaborate with peers to discuss complex cases.

A Living Language

Remember, anatomy, like language, is dynamic. Advances in medical science continually reshape our understanding of the body. For coders, staying informed about these developments isn't just about professional growth—it's about ensuring the accuracy and integrity of the healthcare narrative captured in coded data.

As you navigate the intricate landscape of human anatomy, let your curiosity drive you. Each piece of anatomical knowledge not only makes you a more proficient coder but also deepens your appreciation for the complexity and marvel of the human body.

2.3. Common Medical Conditions and Procedures

Embarking on the journey of medical coding requires familiarity not only with the structure of the human body but also with the various conditions that can affect it and the procedures used to diagnose, treat, or manage these conditions. This section highlights some common medical conditions and procedures you'll encounter as a medical coder, serving as a bridge between the theoretical knowledge of medical terminology and anatomy and the practical application of coding.

Common Medical Conditions

Understanding common medical conditions is crucial for medical coders, as it allows for the accurate interpretation and coding of medical reports. Here's a glimpse into some frequently encountered conditions:

- **Hypertension (High Blood Pressure):** A chronic condition where the force of the blood against the artery walls is too high, often leading to heart disease and stroke.

- **Diabetes Mellitus:** A metabolic disorder characterized by high blood sugar levels over a prolonged period, with Type 1 and Type 2 as the most common forms.

- **Asthma:** A respiratory condition marked by spasms in the bronchi of the lungs, causing difficulty in breathing. It's often linked to allergic reactions or other forms of hypersensitivity.

- **Chronic Obstructive Pulmonary Disease (COPD):** A group of lung diseases that block airflow and make it difficult to breathe, primarily caused by smoking.

- **Osteoarthritis:** A degenerative joint disease caused by the breakdown of joint cartilage and underlying bone, leading to pain and stiffness, especially in the hips, knees, and thumbs.

Common Procedures

In medical coding, you'll frequently encounter documentation of various procedures performed to diagnose, treat, or manage diseases. Familiarity with these procedures and their purposes is essential for accurate coding:

- **Blood Tests:** Including complete blood count (CBC), blood glucose tests, and lipid panels, these tests are fundamental in diagnosing and monitoring various conditions.

- **X-rays:** A form of radiography used to image the inside of the body, especially bones, to diagnose fractures, infections, or tumors.

- **Computed Tomography (CT) Scans:** Advanced imaging technique that provides detailed cross-sectional images of the body, useful in diagnosing diseases or injuries in various body parts.

- **Magnetic Resonance Imaging (MRI):** Uses strong magnetic fields and radio waves to generate detailed images of the organs and tissues in the body, often used for diagnosing brain, spinal cord, and muscle conditions.

- **Biopsies:** Involves the removal of small samples of tissue for examination under a microscope to diagnose cancer or other diseases.

Coding in Context

Accurately coding medical conditions and procedures requires more than just matching symptoms or treatments to codes. It involves understanding the context in which these conditions occur and the rationale behind choosing specific diagnostic or treatment methods. For example, knowing that an MRI is preferred over an X-ray for soft tissue evaluation helps in understanding the medical narrative and ensuring accurate documentation.

Challenges and Strategies

One of the challenges in coding medical conditions and procedures lies in keeping up with advances in medicine that continually introduce new treatments and diagnostic methods. Coders must stay informed through continuous education and by consulting updated coding manuals and resources.

A Lifelong Learning Process

The landscape of common medical conditions and procedures is vast and ever-changing. As a medical coder, your role is not just to code but to understand the evolving nature of healthcare. Engaging with professional coding communities, attending workshops, and leveraging online resources are excellent ways to keep your knowledge current. Remember, each condition and procedure you learn about not only adds to your coding proficiency but also deepens your appreciation for the complexity of human health and the innovative approaches to care.

2.4. Pharmacology Basics for Coders

Pharmacology, the branch of medicine concerned with the uses, effects, and modes of action of drugs, is a critical area for medical coders to understand. While coders are not expected to be pharmacists, a basic grasp of pharmacology enhances the accuracy of coding, especially when dealing with medications in medical reports. This understanding can clarify treatment decisions, help in identifying drug-related procedures, and ensure compliance with coding guidelines related to pharmaceutical treatments.

Understanding Drug Classification

Drugs are categorized based on their effects on the body, their chemical structure, and their therapeutic use. Familiarity with these classifications aids coders in navigating the complexities of medication-related coding. Some broad categories include:

- **Antibiotics:** Used to treat bacterial infections, antibiotics are critical in both acute care and chronic disease management.

- **Analgesics:** Pain relievers, such as acetaminophen and ibuprofen, are common in various treatment plans.

- **Antihypertensives:** These medications control high blood pressure, a common chronic condition.

- **Antidiabetics:** Including insulin and oral hypoglycemics, these drugs manage diabetes mellitus.

- **Statins:** Used to lower cholesterol levels in the blood, statins help in preventing heart disease.

Coding for Medications

When coding for medications, several factors come into play:

- **Generic vs. Brand Names:** Understanding that drugs can be listed under their generic name (the chemical compound) or brand name (given by the manufacturer) is important for accurate documentation.

- **Dosage and Administration:** The route of administration (oral, intravenous, etc.) and dosage can affect coding, especially in scenarios involving medication administration procedures.

- **Drug-Specific Codes:** Certain coding systems, like HCPCS Level II codes in the United States, include codes for drugs and their administration. Familiarity with these codes is essential for billing certain medications and treatments.

Pharmacology in Patient Care

Drugs play a significant role in patient care, serving various functions from treating acute conditions to managing chronic diseases. Coders often encounter medication information in the context of:

- **Treatment Plans:** Medications are a cornerstone of many treatment plans, and understanding their role can provide insights into the patient's condition and care strategy.

- **Adverse Reactions:** Coding for adverse drug reactions requires recognizing the connection between the medication and the patient's symptoms or diagnosis.

- **Medication Reconciliation:** In hospital settings, coding might involve documentation related to reconciling a patient's medications upon admission, during hospitalization, and at discharge.

Challenges and Strategies for Coders

Keeping abreast of new medications and changes to existing drugs presents a challenge due to the dynamic nature of pharmacology. Strategies to stay informed include:

- **Regularly Reviewing Drug Databases:** Online databases and formularies are invaluable resources for up-to-date drug information.

- **Continuing Education:** Pharmacology updates are a staple of medical coding continuing education programs.

- **Collaboration with Healthcare Providers:** When in doubt, consulting with prescribing physicians or pharmacists can clarify uncertainties related to drug coding.

Conclusion

A basic understanding of pharmacology enriches a medical coder's toolkit, enabling more accurate and comprehensive coding of medication-related information. This knowledge supports the broader goal of ensuring that patient care is appropriately documented, coded, and billed, reflecting the complexity and nuances of modern healthcare. As with all aspects of medical coding, curiosity, continuous learning, and collaboration are key to mastering the pharmacological elements of this field.

2.5. Exercise: 10 MCQs with Answers at the End

Test your knowledge on medical terminology, anatomy, common medical conditions and procedures, and pharmacology basics with these multiple-choice questions. Answers are provided at the end to check your understanding.

Questions

1. What does the prefix "hyper-" mean in medical terminology?

   A. Below

   B. Slow

   C. Over, above

   D. Under, beneath

2. Which system of the body is responsible for transporting oxygen and nutrients to the cells?

   A. Respiratory system

   B. Cardiovascular system

   C. Digestive system

   D. Nervous system

3. What is hypertension?

   A. Low blood sugar

   B. High blood pressure

   C. Inflammation of joints

   D. Decreased bone density

4. A CT scan is primarily used to:

A. Measure bone density

B. Examine the soft tissues of the body

C. Record the electrical activity of the heart

D. Test lung function and capacity

5. The medication class known as "statins" is used to:

A. Treat bacterial infections

B. Lower blood pressure

C. Reduce blood sugar levels

D. Lower cholesterol levels

6. Which of the following is a common route of drug administration?

A. Percutaneous

B. Intravenous

C. Transdermal

D. All of the above

7. Diabetes Mellitus affects which system of the body?

A. Muscular system

B. Endocrine system

C. Cardiovascular system

D. Integumentary system

8. Osteoarthritis is a disease affecting the:

A. Heart valves

B. Joints

C. Lungs

D. Brain

9. An MRI is particularly useful for imaging:

A. Bones

B. Soft tissues

C. Blood flow

D. Digestive tract

10. The term "analgesic" refers to medications that:

A. Promote sleep

B. Relieve pain

C. Reduce inflammation

D. Lower fever

Answers

1. C. Over, above

2. B. Cardiovascular system

3. B. High blood pressure

4. B. Examine the soft tissues of the body

5. D. Lower cholesterol levels

6. D. All of the above

7. B. Endocrine system

8. B. Joints

9. B. Soft tissues

10. B. Relieve pain

This exercise is designed to reinforce the foundational knowledge crucial for effective medical coding. Understanding medical terminology, anatomy, common conditions, and pharmacology basics ensures accurate coding and supports the overall healthcare documentation process.

Chapter 3: Introduction to ICD-10

3.1. Understanding ICD-10-CM

The International Classification of Diseases, Tenth Revision, Clinical Modification (ICD-10-CM) is a critical component in the medical coding and billing process, providing a standardized system for classifying diseases and health problems. This coding system is essential for ensuring accurate billing, facilitating epidemiological research, and improving healthcare delivery. Let's delve into the basics of ICD-10-CM, its structure, and its significance in the healthcare industry.

The Evolution of ICD-10-CM

ICD-10-CM is part of a global coding system used for morbidity data. Its predecessor, ICD-9-CM, was replaced due to its limitations in accurately describing modern medical practices and technologies. ICD-10-CM offers a more detailed classification system, accommodating newer diagnoses and procedures, which enhances the accuracy of healthcare data analysis.

Structure of ICD-10-CM

ICD-10-CM codes are alphanumeric and contain 3 to 7 characters. The structure is as follows:

- **First Character:** Alphabetical, indicating the chapter of the classification the condition belongs to.

- **Second and Third Characters:** Numeric, representing the category of the diagnosis.

- **Fourth to Sixth Characters:** These can be alphanumeric and provide details about the etiology, anatomical site, and severity of the condition.

- **Seventh Character:** An extension, used in certain chapters, provides information about the encounter or the phase of treatment.

This structured approach allows for a high level of specificity and detail, facilitating precise coding of patient diagnoses.

Significance in Healthcare

The implementation of ICD-10-CM has several significant implications for healthcare:

- **Improved Accuracy in Billing:** The detailed classification system allows for more precise billing, ensuring that healthcare providers are reimbursed accurately for the services they provide.

- **Enhanced Clinical Documentation:** ICD-10-CM's specificity encourages thorough clinical documentation, which is crucial for patient care, medical research, and healthcare policy-making.

- **Global Standardization:** As part of the global ICD-10 system, ICD-10-CM facilitates the international comparison of healthcare data, contributing to global health research and epidemiological studies.

Challenges and Adaptation

Transitioning from ICD-9-CM to ICD-10-CM presented challenges, primarily due to the need for extensive training and updates to electronic health record (EHR) systems. However, the transition has ultimately led to more accurate and detailed medical records, benefiting healthcare providers, payers, and patients alike.

Coding with ICD-10-CM

Coding accurately with ICD-10-CM requires an understanding of its guidelines, which include conventions, general coding guidelines, and chapter-specific guidelines. Coders must be diligent in keeping up-to-date with annual updates and revisions to the ICD-10-CM system, ensuring the continued accuracy and relevance of the codes used in documentation and billing.

Conclusion

Understanding ICD-10-CM is foundational for medical coders, as it directly impacts billing, healthcare analytics, and the overall management of health information. Its detailed and structured system not only supports the financial aspects of healthcare but also contributes to the quality and continuity of patient care. As healthcare evolves, so too will ICD-10-CM, reflecting the dynamic nature of medicine and the ongoing need for precise and comprehensive healthcare documentation.

3.2. Coding Guidelines for ICD-10

Navigating the complexities of ICD-10-CM requires more than just an understanding of its structure; it demands familiarity with the specific coding guidelines that govern its use. These guidelines ensure consistency, accuracy, and comprehensiveness in coding practices across the healthcare industry. Let's explore the core principles and rules that form the backbone of effective ICD-10-CM coding.

General Coding Guidelines

1. Code to the Highest Level of Specificity: Always use the most detailed code available, ensuring it fully describes the diagnosis or reason for the encounter. This might mean using all available characters in a code, including those that specify laterality or encounter details.

2. Use of Signs and Symptoms: When a definitive diagnosis has not been established, coding signs and symptoms is acceptable. However, once a diagnosis is confirmed, it should be coded instead.

3. Sequencing of Codes: In cases where multiple conditions are present, the primary diagnosis—the condition chiefly responsible for the encounter—should be coded first, followed by secondary diagnoses that provide additional context or are also being managed.

4. Chronic and Acute Conditions: If both an acute and a chronic form of a condition are present, and separate codes exist, both should be coded, with the acute code generally listed first.

5. Coding Guidelines for Outpatient Services: For outpatient services, codes that describe the reason for the encounter (such as symptoms or a confirmed diagnosis) are prioritized. Conditions that were previously treated and no longer exist should not be coded.

Chapter-Specific Guidelines

1. Certain Infectious and Parasitic Diseases (A00-B99): Special attention is given to coding infections, particularly the distinction between sepsis, severe sepsis, and septic shock.

2. Neoplasms (C00-D49): Guidelines specify how to code for primary, secondary, and in situ neoplasms, as well as the treatment of complications associated with malignancies or the treatment thereof.

3. Diseases of the Blood and Blood-Forming Organs (D50-D89): These guidelines address coding for anemias in chronic diseases, neutropenias, and other conditions affecting blood and bone marrow.

4. Endocrine, Nutritional, and Metabolic Diseases (E00-E89): This includes specific rules for diabetes mellitus coding, including the use of insulin, oral hypoglycemics, and injections.

5. Pregnancy, Childbirth, and the Puerperium (O00-O9A): Guidelines here focus on coding for the current episode of care, with specific attention to trimester of pregnancy and the outcome of delivery.

6. External Causes of Morbidity (V00-Y99): These codes provide additional context and are used in conjunction with other codes to provide a complete picture of the patient encounter.

Annual Updates and Revisions

The ICD-10-CM guidelines are subject to annual review and revision, reflecting changes in healthcare diagnosis, treatment, and technology. Coders must stay abreast of these updates to ensure coding practices remain current and accurate.

Conclusion

Adherence to ICD-10-CM coding guidelines is essential for maintaining the integrity of healthcare data, facilitating accurate billing, and ensuring compliance with regulatory standards. These guidelines not only guide coders through the complexities of the coding process but also support the delivery of high-quality patient care by ensuring that health records accurately reflect patient diagnoses and treatments. As the healthcare landscape evolves, so too will these guidelines, requiring coders to engage in continuous learning and professional development.

3.3. Navigating ICD-10-CM Chapter-Specific Guidelines

Delving deeper into the ICD-10-CM, it becomes evident that each chapter not only categorizes diseases and conditions systematically but also comes with its own set of specific guidelines. These chapter-specific guidelines are designed to ensure accurate and effective coding by addressing conditions and situations unique to each section of the ICD-10-CM. Navigating these guidelines is crucial for coders to capture the full scope of a patient's health status. Here's how to adeptly maneuver through these chapter-specific directives.

Understanding the Structure

ICD-10-CM is divided into chapters based on body systems or conditions, such as infectious diseases, neoplasms, and diseases of the circulatory system, among others. Each chapter has unique coding requirements that reflect the intricacies of the diseases and conditions within that category.

Key Areas of Focus

- **Infectious and Parasitic Diseases (Chapter 1):** This includes guidelines on coding for HIV, sepsis, and other infections, emphasizing the importance of distinguishing between causative agents and the diseases they cause.

- **Neoplasms (Chapter 2):** Guidelines here instruct on coding primary, secondary, in situ, and benign neoplasms, as well as coding for patients receiving treatment for malignancies.

- **Diseases of the Blood and Blood-Forming Organs (Chapter 3):** Specific instructions are provided for coding anemias, hemoglobinopathies, and other hematologic conditions, focusing on the underlying cause or type of anemia.

- **Endocrine, Nutritional, and Metabolic Diseases (Chapter 4):** This includes detailed guidelines on coding diabetes mellitus, obesity, malnutrition, and thyroid disorders, with an emphasis on associated complications and controlled/uncontrolled status.

- **Mental, Behavioral, and Neurodevelopmental Disorders (Chapter 5):** Coders are guided on how to document conditions like depression, schizophrenia, and autism spectrum disorders, considering the significance of episode recurrences and severity.

- **Diseases of the Nervous System (Chapter 6):** Guidelines cover a range of conditions from epilepsy to Alzheimer's disease, focusing on specificity regarding causation and manifestations.

- **Diseases of the Eye and Adnexa (Chapter 7) and Diseases of the Ear and Mastoid Process (Chapter 8):** These sections emphasize the coding of laterality and the stage or severity of conditions.

- **Pregnancy, Childbirth, and the Puerperium (Chapter 15):** Coders are instructed to use codes from this chapter for the primary diagnosis in cases related to pregnancy, with detailed guidelines on trimester coding and complications.

Strategies for Navigating Chapter-Specific Guidelines

1. **Stay Informed:** Regularly review updates to the ICD-10-CM, including changes to chapter-specific guidelines, which are updated annually.

2. **Use Reliable Resources:** Leverage official coding manuals, online resources, and professional forums to understand and apply these guidelines effectively.

3. **Practice Scenario-Based Learning:** Engage with coding scenarios and case studies that apply chapter-specific guidelines to solidify understanding and application skills.

4. **Seek Clarification:** When in doubt, consult with more experienced coders, coding auditors, or healthcare providers to ensure accurate coding decisions.

5. **Continuous Education:** Participate in coding workshops, webinars, and continuing education courses focused on ICD-10-CM coding to stay current with best practices.

Conclusion

Navigating the chapter-specific guidelines of ICD-10-CM is a fundamental skill for medical coders, ensuring that every aspect of a patient's condition is accurately captured and coded. This not only facilitates appropriate reimbursement but also contributes to the quality of patient care and the advancement of medical research. Through diligent study, ongoing education, and practical application, coders can master these guidelines, enhancing their proficiency and accuracy in medical coding.

3.4. Common ICD-10 Coding Challenges

Transitioning to and navigating the ICD-10-CM coding system, while beneficial for its specificity and accuracy, has introduced a variety of challenges for medical coders. These challenges can impact billing, compliance, and even patient care if not addressed properly. Understanding these common hurdles is the first step in overcoming them. Here are some of the most prevalent ICD-10 coding challenges and strategies for managing them effectively.

1. Increased Specificity and Detail

One of the most significant changes with ICD-10-CM is the level of detail and specificity required in coding diagnoses. While this allows for more accurate data capture, it also requires coders to have a comprehensive understanding of medical terminology, anatomy, and the conditions being coded.

- **Strategy:** Enhance your knowledge base through continuous education and use of detailed clinical documentation to make the most accurate coding decisions.

2. Documentation Gaps

The specificity of ICD-10-CM often highlights inadequacies in clinical documentation, making it difficult for coders to assign the most accurate codes. This gap can lead to queries to providers and delays in coding.

- **Strategy:** Work closely with healthcare providers to improve the quality of clinical documentation. Implementing regular training sessions for providers on the importance of detailed documentation can also help bridge this gap.

3. Keeping Up with Code Updates

ICD-10-CM codes are updated annually, introducing new codes, deleting obsolete ones, and revising existing codes. Staying current with these changes is crucial for accurate coding and billing.

- **Strategy:** Make a habit of reviewing the annual updates to ICD-10-CM as soon as they are released. Utilize resources from the CDC and WHO, as well as professional coding organizations, to stay informed.

4. Sequencing and Coding Guidelines

Proper code sequencing is essential in ICD-10-CM, especially when dealing with multiple diagnoses. Understanding and applying the coding guidelines correctly is crucial for accurate reimbursement and data reporting.

- **Strategy:** Regularly review the official ICD-10-CM coding guidelines and participate in coding seminars and workshops focused on sequencing and guideline application.

5. Use of Unspecified Codes

While ICD-10-CM aims for specificity, there are instances where coders may resort to using unspecified codes, which can lead to issues with reimbursement and data quality.

- **Strategy:** Only use unspecified codes when absolutely necessary and after all other resources have been exhausted. Encourage clinicians to provide as much detail as possible in their documentation.

6. External Cause Codes

The correct use of external cause codes can be confusing, especially determining when and how they should be applied to fully capture the details of an encounter.

- **Strategy:** Develop a clear understanding of the purpose and application of external cause codes through guidelines and training. Use these codes to complement the diagnosis codes for a complete picture of the encounter.

7. Coding for Comorbidities and Complications

Identifying and coding comorbidities and complications requires a deep understanding of how these conditions interact and affect patient care and outcomes.

- **Strategy:** Focus on comprehensive education regarding diseases and conditions, emphasizing the relationships between comorbidities and primary conditions. Use case studies and real-life scenarios to practice coding for complex cases.

Conclusion

While ICD-10-CM presents a variety of coding challenges, effectively navigating these obstacles is possible through continuous education, collaboration with healthcare providers, and a deep understanding of the coding system. Embracing these challenges as opportunities for growth can enhance coding accuracy, improve healthcare data quality, and contribute to better patient outcomes.

3.5. Exercise: 10 MCQs with Answers at the End

Test your understanding of the intricacies of ICD-10-CM with these multiple-choice questions. They cover a range of topics from the introduction to ICD-10-CM, coding guidelines, navigating chapter-specific guidelines, to common coding challenges. Answers are provided at the end for self-assessment.

Questions

1. ICD-10-CM stands for:

   A. International Classification of Diseases, 10th Modification

   B. International Codification of Diseases, 10th Correction

   C. International Classification of Diseases, 10th Revision, Clinical Modification

   D. International Catalog of Diseases, 10th Revision, Clinical Modification

2. The first character in an ICD-10-CM code is always:

   A. Numeric

   B. Alphanumeric

   C. A letter

   D. A symbol

3. When coding with ICD-10-CM, if both acute and chronic conditions are present, how should they be coded?

A. Only the acute condition is coded

B. Only the chronic condition is coded

C. The acute condition is listed first

D. The chronic condition is listed first

4. Which update frequency does ICD-10-CM follow?

A. Biennial

B. Quarterly

C. Annually

D. Semi-annually

5. For outpatient coding, the primary diagnosis is:

A. The most severe diagnosis

B. The diagnosis that prompted the hospital admission

C. The reason for the encounter as stated by the physician

D. Always a chronic condition

6. Sequencing of ICD-10-CM codes is important because:

A. It determines the primary focus of treatment

B. It affects reimbursement rates

C. It can impact patient outcomes

D. Both A and B are correct

7. An unspecified code in ICD-10-CM should be used:

A. As a first choice when documentation is lacking

B. When there is not enough information to code more specifically

C. Frequently, to save time

D. Never, under any circumstances

8. External cause codes in ICD-10-CM are used to:

A. Replace diagnosis codes

B. Supplement the diagnosis codes with additional detail

C. Code psychological conditions

D. Indicate the primary diagnosis

9. Which of the following best describes the annual updates to ICD-10-CM?

A. Introduction of new diseases only

B. Revisions to coding guidelines and addition or deletion of codes

C. Changes to the alphabetical index only

D. Updates to the tabular list of diseases only

10. The greatest challenge in transitioning to ICD-10-CM was:

    A. The increase in the number of codes

    B. Learning to use electronic health records

    C. The specificity and detail required in documentation

    D. The need to recode all past medical records

Answers

1. C. International Classification of Diseases, 10th Revision, Clinical Modification

2. C. A letter

3. C. The acute condition is listed first

4. C. Annually

5. C. The reason for the encounter as stated by the physician

6. D. Both A and B are correct

7. B. When there is not enough information to code more specifically

8. B. Supplement the diagnosis codes with additional detail

9. B. Revisions to coding guidelines and addition or deletion of codes

10. C. The specificity and detail required in documentation

These questions and answers are designed to reinforce key concepts of ICD-10-CM coding and address common areas of confusion, helping coders to navigate the complexities of the system more effectively.

Chapter 4: Advanced ICD-10 Coding

4.1. Complex Case Studies in ICD-10

Mastering ICD-10 coding requires more than understanding the basics; it involves navigating complex case studies that reflect the multifaceted nature of healthcare diagnoses and treatments. These complex case studies challenge coders to apply their knowledge, analytical skills, and attention to detail to ensure accurate and comprehensive coding. Here, we explore how to approach complex case studies in ICD-10, highlighting the strategies for dealing with nuanced coding scenarios.

Approach to Complex Cases

1. **Thorough Review of Documentation:** Start by reviewing all available medical documentation to understand the patient's condition fully. This includes physician notes, surgical reports, diagnostic findings, and treatment plans. A comprehensive review ensures you don't miss any critical information that could impact coding.

2. **Identify Primary and Secondary Conditions:** Determine the primary diagnosis that led to the patient's encounter, followed by any secondary conditions that also require attention.

Remember, the sequencing of these diagnoses can affect reimbursement and reflects the patient's clinical picture.

3. **Apply ICD-10 Guidelines:** Use the ICD-10-CM guidelines to navigate coding for specific conditions, particularly those that have specific rules, such as injuries, poisonings, and certain chronic diseases. Pay close attention to chapter-specific guidelines for conditions that fall under multiple categories.

4. **Consider External Cause Codes:** For cases involving injuries or external factors, include external cause codes to provide additional context about the circumstances of the injury or condition. These codes are crucial for injury-related encounters and can provide valuable data for public health monitoring.

5. **Utilize Combination Codes:** ICD-10-CM includes many combination codes that describe a condition and its common symptoms or manifestations in one code. Identifying and using these codes when appropriate can streamline the coding process and reduce errors.

6. **Check for Laterality and Specificity:** Many ICD-10 codes require information on laterality (left, right, bilateral) and specify the condition's stage or severity. Ensure that the codes you select convey this information when applicable.

Strategies for Complex Coding Challenges

- **Coding for Comorbidities:** When patients present with multiple chronic conditions, each affecting the patient's health status, coders must carefully document all relevant diagnoses, ensuring they reflect the patient's clinical complexity.

- **Postoperative Complications:** Coding for postoperative complications requires coders to discern whether a symptom is a routine post-surgical occurrence or a complication that affects the course of treatment.

- **Chronic Disease Exacerbations:** Episodes where a chronic disease worsens pose coding challenges, especially in distinguishing between routine management of a chronic condition and treatment for an exacerbation.

Example Case Study

Consider a patient admitted with acute respiratory failure due to severe COPD exacerbation, with a history of hypertension and type 2 diabetes. The patient also suffers from a postoperative wound infection following a recent knee replacement.

- **Primary Diagnosis:** Acute respiratory failure (J96.0x)

- **Secondary Diagnoses:** COPD exacerbation (J44.1), hypertension (I10), type 2 diabetes (E11.-), postoperative wound infection (T81.4xx)

- **Procedure Codes:** Include codes for any treatments or diagnostic procedures performed specifically for the exacerbation or complications.

Conclusion

Complex case studies in ICD-10 coding demand a nuanced approach, where coders must balance the specificity of coding requirements with the clinical picture presented by the patient. Through meticulous documentation review, adherence to ICD-10 guidelines, and a detailed understanding of the patient's conditions and treatments, coders can navigate these challenges effectively. Continuous learning and staying updated with ICD-10-CM changes are essential for success in coding complex cases.

4.2. ICD-10-CM Coding for Specialized Areas

Specialized areas of medicine often require a deep understanding of specific ICD-10-CM coding guidelines, reflecting the unique challenges and nuances of coding for complex conditions and treatments. From oncology to obstetrics, each area demands a focused approach to accurately capture the clinical picture. Here's a look at strategies and considerations for ICD-10-CM coding in several specialized medical fields.

Oncology

Coding for oncology involves understanding the classification of neoplasms and the specifics of coding for primary, secondary, and in situ cancers. It's crucial to accurately document the type, location, and behavior of the tumor, as well as treatment methods like chemotherapy, radiation, and surgery.

- **Key Considerations:** Pay attention to codes for personal history of cancer (Z85.-), which can impact patient care plans and surveillance strategies. Also, the distinction between active treatment and palliative care is critical for accurate coding.

Obstetrics

Obstetrics coding covers a wide range of conditions related to pregnancy, childbirth, and the postpartum period. This includes coding for routine prenatal visits, complications of pregnancy, labor and delivery, and the postpartum condition of the mother.

- **Key Considerations:** The use of trimester-specific codes and the outcome of delivery code (Z37.-) are essential. Coding for the perinatal period requires special attention to the transition from intrauterine to extrauterine life, with specific codes for conditions originating in the perinatal period (P00-P96).

Pediatrics

Pediatric coding must account for conditions that are congenital, developmental, or acquired during childhood. This includes a wide range of conditions from congenital anomalies (Q00-Q99) to developmental disorders and common pediatric illnesses.

- **Key Considerations:** Many pediatric codes require specificity regarding age, as certain conditions are coded differently in children than in adults. Additionally, documentation of growth and development milestones can impact coding decisions.

Psychiatry

Psychiatric coding involves the use of codes for mental, behavioral, and neurodevelopmental disorders (F01-F99). This includes coding for conditions such as depression, anxiety, bipolar disorder, and schizophrenia.

- **Key Considerations:** The severity, episode recurrences, and the presence of psychotic features are important for accurate coding. Substance use disorders require codes that specify the substance and the nature of the use (abuse, dependence).

Neurology

Coding for neurological conditions involves a range of disorders from epilepsy (G40.-) to Alzheimer's disease (G30.-). It requires detailed documentation of the condition's type, severity, and progression.

- **Key Considerations:** For conditions like stroke (I60-I69), coding must reflect the type of stroke, the affected vessel, and the presence of any sequelae. Similarly, codes for epilepsies and seizures are specific to the type and intractability of the seizures.

Strategies for Specialized Coding

1. **Continuous Education:** Stay updated with the latest coding guidelines and changes specific to your area of specialization through webinars, workshops, and certification courses.

2. **Detailed Documentation:** Work closely with healthcare providers to ensure documentation is comprehensive, covering all aspects of the patient's condition and treatment.

3. **Use of Clinical Resources:** Leverage clinical decision support tools and resources to understand complex conditions better and ensure accurate coding.

4. **Peer Collaboration:** Engage with peers in specialized coding areas to share knowledge, discuss challenging cases, and stay informed about best practices.

Conclusion

Coding for specialized areas in ICD-10-CM demands a nuanced understanding of both the medical conditions specific to the field and the detailed coding guidelines that apply. By focusing on continuous education, detailed documentation, and collaboration, coders can navigate the complexities of specialized coding, ensuring accuracy and contributing to high-quality patient care.

4.3. Using the ICD-10-CM Index and Tabular List

Navigating the ICD-10-CM requires proficiency in using both the Alphabetic Index and the Tabular List effectively. These two components are essential tools for medical coders, allowing for the accurate and efficient identification of codes based on diagnoses, symptoms, or conditions documented in patient records. Understanding how to use these resources is key to mastering ICD-10-CM coding.

The Alphabetic Index

The Alphabetic Index is divided into several sections, including the Index to Diseases and Injuries, the Table of Neoplasms, and the Index to External Causes of Injury. It's the starting point for finding a code, guiding coders from a known condition or term to a preliminary code.

- **Approach:** Begin by looking up the main term, which is typically the condition, symptom, or diagnosis. Subterms under the main term can provide more specificity, leading to a more precise code. It's crucial to review all relevant subterms and cross-references, as they may direct you to different coding options.

- **Tips for Using the Index:**

  - Always cross-reference subterms and consider modifiers that may affect code selection.

  - Pay attention to "see" and "see also" references, which guide you to the most accurate coding path.

  - Utilize the Table of Neoplasms and the Index to External Causes when coding for cancers and injuries, respectively, to find appropriate codes based on the nature and cause of the condition.

The Tabular List

The Tabular List is a structured list of ICD-10-CM codes divided by chapters based on disease type or body system. Each code is accompanied by a description and may include inclusion and exclusion notes, coding guidelines, and instructions for use.

- **Approach:** After identifying a preliminary code in the Index, verify it in the Tabular List. This step is crucial for confirming the accuracy of the code, understanding any additional coding instructions, and ensuring that the code is the most specific option available.

- **Tips for Using the Tabular List:**

 - Read the complete code description and any applicable inclusion or exclusion notes to ensure the selected code fully captures the documented condition.

 - Look for instructions on additional codes required for certain conditions, such as etiology/manifestation pairings.

 - Be aware of codes that require a seventh character for episode of care or other specific details, ensuring the code is complete.

Common Challenges and Solutions

- **Finding Specific Conditions:** Conditions documented in patient records may not always match terms exactly as listed in the Index. It may be necessary to consider synonyms or clinical equivalents.

- **Solution:** Use clinical knowledge and available resources to determine the most accurate term for lookup. Collaboration with clinical staff may also provide clarity.

- **Choosing Between Similar Codes:** The Index may guide you to multiple codes that seem applicable.

- **Solution:** Use the Tabular List to read the full descriptions and guidelines for each code, choosing the one that best matches the documented condition based on specificity and clinical documentation.

- **Sequencing and Additional Codes:** Determining the correct sequence of codes or when additional codes are needed can be challenging.

- **Solution:** Refer to the official coding guidelines and any chapter-specific instructions in the Tabular List to understand sequencing rules and the requirement for additional codes.

Conclusion

Mastering the use of the ICD-10-CM Index and Tabular List is fundamental to accurate medical coding. By starting with the Index for initial code identification and then verifying and refining the selection with the Tabular List, coders can ensure that they capture the full scope of the patient's condition accurately and comprehensively. Continuous practice, along with a solid understanding of medical terminology and clinical concepts, will enhance proficiency in using these essential coding tools.

4.4. ICD-10-CM Updates and Changes

Staying abreast of annual updates and changes to the ICD-10-CM is crucial for medical coders, healthcare providers, and billing professionals. These updates can include the addition, deletion, or revision of codes, along with changes to coding guidelines that reflect advances in medical knowledge, public health trends, and the healthcare industry's evolving needs. Understanding and incorporating these changes into coding practices ensures accurate billing, compliance, and the effective tracking of health trends.

Nature of ICD-10-CM Updates

1. **Addition of New Codes:** New diseases, emerging health issues, and advancements in medical technology can lead to the addition of new codes, allowing for more precise documentation of healthcare encounters.

2. **Deletion of Codes:** Codes can be deleted when they become obsolete, redundant, or are consolidated into new, more specific codes. This process ensures the coding system remains efficient and relevant.

3. **Revision of Existing Codes:** Revisions might involve changes to code descriptions, instructional notes, or the reclassification of conditions to more appropriate categories. These adjustments improve the accuracy and clarity of coding.

Impact of Updates on Coding Practices

- **Clinical Documentation:** Updates can necessitate more detailed clinical documentation to support the use of new or revised codes, emphasizing the need for ongoing education for healthcare providers.

- **Billing and Reimbursement:** Changes in codes can affect reimbursement rates and billing processes, requiring adjustments in billing practices to ensure compliance and optimize revenue cycle management.

- **Public Health Reporting:** The introduction of new codes, especially for emerging diseases or public health concerns, is essential for tracking health trends, resource allocation, and policy planning at the national and global levels.

Strategies for Managing ICD-10-CM Updates

1. **Annual Training:** Coders and healthcare professionals should participate in annual training sessions focused on the latest ICD-10-CM updates to ensure they are coding accurately and effectively.

2. **Utilize Official Resources:** The Centers for Disease Control and Prevention (CDC) and the World Health Organization (WHO) provide resources and tools to help understand and implement code changes.

3. **Update Coding Manuals and Software:** Ensure that coding manuals, electronic health record (EHR) systems, and billing software are updated to reflect the latest codes and guidelines.

4. **Practice Coding with New Codes:** Engage in practice coding exercises that incorporate new codes and scenarios to build familiarity and confidence with the updates.

5. **Monitor Coding Quality:** Implement quality control measures to monitor the accuracy of coding with the new updates, identifying areas where additional training or resources may be needed.

Conclusion

The dynamic nature of ICD-10-CM requires coders to be adaptable, informed, and proactive in integrating annual updates into their coding practices. By understanding the rationale behind changes, leveraging available resources, and prioritizing education and quality control, coders can effectively navigate updates, contributing to the integrity of health data and the broader goals of healthcare quality, billing accuracy, and public health surveillance.

4.5. Exercise: 10 MCQs with Answers at the End

Challenge your knowledge on the advanced aspects of ICD-10 coding, including complex case studies, specialized areas, the use of the Index and Tabular List, and staying updated with ICD-10-CM changes. Review these multiple-choice questions to reinforce your understanding. Answers are provided for self-assessment.

Questions

1. What is the primary purpose of annual updates to the ICD-10-CM?

   A. To correct spelling errors in the manual

 B. To add, delete, or revise codes based on new medical knowledge and technologies

   C. To increase the complexity of the coding system

D. To change the structure of the coding system annually

2. In oncology coding, what is essential to specify when coding for neoplasms?

A. The patient's age and gender

B. The size of the tumor only

C. The behavior, site, and morphology of the neoplasm

D. The number of tumors present

3. When using the ICD-10-CM Index, what should you do if directed by a "see also" note?

A. Ignore the note as it is usually optional

B. Consult the Tabular List immediately without following the note

C. Follow the note for additional instructions or options

D. Only use the original code found, not the one referenced in the note

4. Which of the following best describes the use of external cause codes in ICD-10-CM?

A. They are primary codes that replace diagnosis codes

B. They are used only when no other codes are applicable

C. They provide additional detail about the circumstances of an injury or health condition

D. They are mandatory for all injury-related diagnoses

5. For coding in obstetrics, how are trimester-specific codes determined?

A. By the baby's weight at birth

B. By the gestational age documented in the medical record

C. By the mother's age

D. By the number of fetuses

6. What is a key consideration when coding psychiatric conditions in ICD-10-CM?

A. The phase of the moon at the time of diagnosis

B. The severity and recurrence of the condition

C. The patient's family history only

D. The medication prescribed to the patient

7. When are unspecified codes in ICD-10-CM appropriate to use?

A. When specific information is not available for a more precise code

B. As the first choice to save time

C. To avoid looking up specific codes

D. When the coder is unsure about the correct code

8. How should chronic diseases that are stable and require no treatment be coded?

A. They should not be coded

B. As active conditions

C. With an unspecified code

D. As historical conditions, if they impact the current care or treatment

9. In the context of ICD-10-CM, what does a combination code allow a coder to do?

A. Code multiple unrelated diagnoses with a single code

B. Report a diagnosis and its common manifestation or complication in one code

C. Combine procedure codes with diagnosis codes

D. Use a single code to capture all of a patient's chronic conditions

10. The Tabular List in ICD-10-CM is used for:

A. Finding the initial code based on a diagnosis description

B. Verifying the code found in the Index and reviewing any applicable instructions

C. Looking up medications related to a diagnosis

D. Determining the patient's prognosis

Answers

1. B. To add, delete, or revise codes based on new medical knowledge and technologies

2. C. The behavior, site, and morphology of the neoplasm

3. C. Follow the note for additional instructions or options

4. C. They provide additional detail about the circumstances of an injury or health condition

5. B. By the gestational age documented in the medical record

6. B. The severity and recurrence of the condition

7. A. When specific information is not available for a more precise code

8. D. As historical conditions, if they impact the current care or treatment

9. B. Report a diagnosis and its common manifestation or complication in one code

10. B. Verifying the code found in the Index and reviewing any applicable instructions

These questions are designed to deepen your understanding of advanced ICD-10 coding practices, emphasizing the importance of accuracy, specificity, and adherence to updated guidelines in medical coding.

Chapter 5: Introduction to CPT and HCPCS

5.1. Understanding CPT Coding System

The Current Procedural Terminology (CPT) coding system is a comprehensive and standardized set of codes used by physicians, allied health professionals, and healthcare providers to report medical, surgical, and diagnostic procedures and services. Developed and maintained by the American Medical Association (AMA), the CPT coding system plays a crucial role in the healthcare billing process, facilitating the accurate description of medical services and procedures for reimbursement from insurance companies and government payers.

Components of the CPT Coding System

CPT codes are divided into three categories, each serving a specific purpose:

- **Category I:** The most widely used set of codes, representing procedures and services that are widely performed and accepted in clinical practice. These codes are five-digit numeric codes organized into six sections: Evaluation and Management,

Anesthesiology, Surgery, Radiology, Pathology and Laboratory, and Medicine.

- **Category II:** These are supplemental tracking codes used for performance management. They offer a way to collect information about the quality of care provided. These codes are not used for billing but rather for data collection and performance improvement.

- **Category III:** These codes represent emerging technologies, services, and procedures. They allow for the tracking and analysis of new procedures and services, providing a mechanism for their potential inclusion in Category I upon becoming widely accepted in clinical practice.

Using CPT Codes

The accurate selection of CPT codes is essential for:

- **Billing and Reimbursement:** Ensuring that healthcare providers are reimbursed for the services they provide. Accurate coding minimizes claim denials and delays.

- **Standardization:** CPT codes offer a standardized language for describing healthcare services, facilitating communication among providers, payers, and administrators.

- **Data Analysis and Research:** The use of standardized codes allows for the analysis of healthcare trends, the efficacy of treatments, and the management of healthcare resources.

Key Considerations in CPT Coding

- **Specificity and Documentation:** The selection of the correct CPT code requires detailed documentation that clearly describes the services provided. Documentation must support the code chosen to avoid denials for lack of medical necessity.

- **Modifiers:** CPT modifiers are used to provide additional information about the performed procedure or service. They can indicate that a service or procedure has been altered in some way without changing its definition.

- **Staying Updated:** The CPT coding system is updated annually to reflect advances in medical technology and the introduction of new procedures. Staying informed about these updates is critical for accurate coding.

Challenges in CPT Coding

CPT coding can present challenges, including keeping up with annual updates, understanding when and how to use modifiers correctly, and ensuring comprehensive documentation to support the codes billed. Continuous education and the use of authoritative resources are essential for overcoming these challenges.

Conclusion

Understanding the CPT coding system is foundational for medical coders, healthcare providers, and billing professionals. It not only facilitates accurate billing and reimbursement but also contributes to the broader goals of healthcare management, including quality assessment, research, and policy development. Mastery of CPT coding requires ongoing education, attention to detail, and a thorough understanding of medical procedures and services.

5.2. Basics of HCPCS Level II

The Healthcare Common Procedure Coding System (HCPCS) Level II is a standardized coding system used alongside the Current Procedural Terminology (CPT) codes. It is used primarily to identify products, supplies, and services not included in the CPT codes, such as ambulance services, durable medical equipment (DME), prosthetics, orthotics, and other medical supplies and services used outside of a physician's office. Managed by the Centers for Medicare & Medicaid Services (CMS), HCPCS Level II codes are essential for billing Medicare and Medicaid claims, and they are widely used by private insurers as well.

Structure of HCPCS Level II Codes

HCPCS Level II codes are alphanumeric, consisting of a single letter followed by four digits, which categorize the types of items or services provided. These codes are organized into the following major groups, each identified by the initial letter:

- **A codes (A0000-A9999):** Transportation, Medical & Surgical Supplies, Miscellaneous & Experimental

- **B codes (B0000-B9999):** Enteral and Parenteral Therapy

- **C codes (C0000-C9999):** Temporary Hospital Outpatient Prospective Payment System

- **D codes (D0000-D9999):** Dental Procedures

- **E codes (E0000-E9999):** Durable Medical Equipment

- **G codes (G0000-G9999):** Temporary Procedures & Professional Services

- **H codes (H0000-H9999):** Rehabilitative Services

- **J codes (J0000-J9999):** Drugs Administered Other Than Oral Method, Chemotherapy Drugs

- **K codes (K0000-K9999):** Temporary Codes for Durable Medical Equipment Regional Carriers

- **L codes (L0000-L9999):** Orthotic and Prosthetic Procedures

- **M codes (M0000-M9999):** Medical Services

- **P codes (P0000-P9999):** Pathology and Laboratory

- **Q codes (Q0000-Q9999):** Temporary Codes

- **R codes (R0000-R9999):** Radiology Services

- **S codes (S0000-S9999):** Commercial Payers

- **T codes (T0000-T9999):** State Medicaid Agency Codes

- **V codes (V0000-V9999):** Vision, Hearing, and Speech-Language Pathology Services

Using HCPCS Level II Codes

For billing and claims processing, HCPCS Level II codes are used to report specific medical items or services not covered by CPT codes. This includes:

- **Medicare and Medicaid Claims:** HCPCS Level II codes are critical for reimbursement for services and supplies under these programs.

- **Private Insurance:** Many private insurers also require the use of HCPCS Level II codes for the billing of drugs, supplies, and certain services.

Key Considerations in HCPCS Level II Coding

- **Accuracy and Documentation:** Accurate coding requires thorough documentation that supports the use of the selected HCPCS Level II code, detailing the necessity and use of the item or service provided.

- **Modifiers:** Similar to CPT codes, HCPCS Level II codes can be modified to further describe the circumstances of the service or item provided. Understanding how to correctly apply these modifiers is essential for accurate billing.

- **Annual Updates:** HCPCS Level II codes are updated annually, with new codes added, and obsolete codes deleted or revised. Staying current with these updates is vital for maintaining billing accuracy and compliance.

Challenges and Strategies

Navigating HCPCS Level II coding involves staying informed about annual updates, understanding the nuances of modifiers, and ensuring that documentation supports the codes used. Coders and billing professionals must:

- **Engage in Continuous Learning:** Regularly participate in training and professional development opportunities to stay updated on HCPCS Level II coding changes and guidelines.

- **Utilize Official Resources:** CMS and other authoritative sources provide guidance, updates, and resources to help professionals accurately apply HCPCS Level II codes.

- **Collaborate with Healthcare Providers:** Work closely with providers to ensure that documentation accurately reflects the services and supplies for which reimbursement is sought.

Conclusion

HCPCS Level II codes play a crucial role in the healthcare billing process, enabling the accurate and standardized reporting of a wide range of services and supplies. Mastery of these codes, alongside CPT coding, is essential for medical coders and billing professionals to ensure effective reimbursement practices and compliance with payer requirements.

5.3. CPT Modifiers and Their Use

CPT modifiers are two-digit numeric or alphanumeric codes added to a CPT code to provide additional information about the medical service or procedure performed. Modifiers help convey specific circumstances that affect a service without changing the definition of the underlying procedure. Their correct use is crucial for accurate billing, ensuring that healthcare providers are reimbursed appropriately while avoiding issues of overcoding or undercoding.

Purpose of CPT Modifiers

Modifiers are used to indicate that:

- A service or procedure has been altered in some way without changing its definition.

- Only a part of the service was performed.

- An adjunctive service was performed in conjunction with another procedure.

- Specific circumstances apply to the service provided that may affect reimbursement.

Commonly Used CPT Modifiers

Some widely used modifiers and their purposes include:

- **Modifier -25:** Significant, Separately Identifiable Evaluation and Management Service by the Same Physician on the Same Day of the Procedure or Other Service. It indicates that a patient's condition required a significant, separately identifiable E/M service beyond the usual pre- and post-operative care associated with the procedure code.

- **Modifier -50:** Bilateral Procedure. This is used when a procedure performed on both sides of the body is reported on a single claim line.

- **Modifier -59:** Distinct Procedural Service. It signifies that a procedure or service was distinct or independent from other services performed on the same day.

- **Modifier -26:** Professional Component. This indicates that only the professional component of the service was provided, such as interpretation of a diagnostic test.

- **Modifier -TC:** Technical Component. It signifies that only the technical portion of the service was performed, such as the provision of equipment or technical staff.

Guidelines for Using Modifiers

- **Documentation:** Adequate documentation must support the use of modifiers. Medical records should clearly justify why a modifier is necessary.

- **Correct Pairing:** Modifiers must be correctly paired with the CPT codes they modify. Misuse can lead to claim denials or incorrect reimbursement.

- **Compliance with Payer Policies:** Familiarity with specific payer policies regarding modifier use is essential, as requirements can vary.

Challenges and Solutions

- **Overuse or Misuse:** Incorrect application of modifiers can lead to claim denials or audits. Solution: Coders should undergo regular training and have access to up-to-date coding resources and guidelines.

- **Documentation Gaps:** Lack of proper documentation supporting the use of modifiers is a common issue. Solution: Work closely with healthcare providers to ensure that documentation is thorough and justifies the use of modifiers.

- **Staying Informed:** Keeping up with changes to modifier definitions and guidelines can be challenging. Solution: Engage in continuous education and utilize authoritative sources like the AMA and CMS for the latest updates.

Conclusion

CPT modifiers play a critical role in medical coding and billing, providing a mechanism to accurately describe the complexity and nature of services rendered. Correct use of modifiers ensures precise communication with payers, facilitating appropriate reimbursement and minimizing the risk of claim denials. Continuous education, proper documentation, and adherence to coding guidelines are essential for effective modifier application.

5.4. Common CPT and HCPCS Coding Scenarios

Navigating the complexities of CPT (Current Procedural Terminology) and HCPCS (Healthcare Common Procedure Coding System) codes requires understanding how to apply them in various clinical scenarios. These coding systems are essential for documenting medical, surgical, and diagnostic services, ensuring accurate billing and reimbursement. Below, we explore common scenarios that highlight the practical application of CPT and HCPCS codes.

Scenario 1: Office Visits and Evaluation & Management (E/M) Services

A patient visits their primary care physician for a comprehensive evaluation of chronic conditions including hypertension and diabetes.

- **CPT Coding:** The visit may be coded using E/M codes (99201-99215), which reflect the complexity and time spent on the patient's care. The use of modifier -25 might be necessary if a significant, separately identifiable E/M service is provided on the same day as another procedure or service.

Scenario 2: Surgical Procedures and Modifiers

A patient undergoes a bilateral carpal tunnel release surgery in an outpatient surgical center.

- **CPT Coding:** The procedure would be reported with the code for carpal tunnel release (e.g., 64721) along with modifier -50 to indicate a bilateral procedure. The facility fee might be billed using HCPCS Level II codes.

Scenario 3: Diagnostic Tests and Technical/Professional Components

A radiology center performs an MRI of the brain, and the radiologist provides the interpretation.

- **CPT Coding:** The MRI procedure might be reported with a code like 70551. Modifiers -TC (Technical Component) and -26 (Professional Component) would be used to differentiate the technical aspect of providing the MRI from the professional interpretation by the radiologist.

Scenario 4: Durable Medical Equipment (DME)

A patient with severe osteoarthritis is prescribed a knee brace by their orthopedic surgeon.

- **HCPCS Coding:** The knee brace would be coded using an appropriate HCPCS Level II code (e.g., L1832) to indicate the specific type of brace provided.

Scenario 5: Administration of Medications

A patient receives an intravenous chemotherapy infusion for cancer treatment at an oncology clinic.

- **HCPCS Coding:** The drug administered would be reported using a specific HCPCS Level II code (e.g., J9000 for Doxorubicin), while the administration of the drug might be captured with CPT codes (e.g., 96413 for chemotherapy administration, intravenous infusion up to 1 hour).

Scenario 6: Use of Modifiers for Special Circumstances

During an outpatient visit, a patient receives multiple services including an E/M service, a minor surgical procedure, and a separate diagnostic procedure.

- **CPT Coding:** Each service would be coded separately, using the appropriate CPT codes. Modifiers such as -25 (for the E/M service that is significant and separately identifiable from the procedures performed) and -59 (to indicate a distinct procedural service) may be necessary to accurately reflect the services provided.

Key Considerations for Coding Scenarios

- **Accuracy and Specificity:** Select codes that most accurately describe the services provided, using modifiers where appropriate to provide additional detail.

- **Documentation:** Ensure that medical records adequately support the codes selected, including the use of modifiers.

- **Compliance:** Stay informed of coding guidelines and payer policies to ensure compliance and optimize reimbursement.

Conclusion

Effective CPT and HCPCS coding is pivotal for accurate billing and reimbursement in healthcare. By understanding how to apply these codes in common clinical scenarios, coders can ensure that medical services are accurately documented and billed, reflecting the care provided to patients. Continuous education and adherence to current coding standards are essential for maintaining coding accuracy and compliance.

5.5. Exercise: 10 MCQs with Answers at the End

Test your knowledge on the basics of CPT and HCPCS coding systems, their application in medical billing, and understanding of modifiers and coding scenarios. Answers are provided at the end for self-assessment.

Questions

1. What is the primary purpose of CPT codes?

   A. To track inventory in healthcare facilities

   B. To report medical, surgical, and diagnostic services for billing

   C. To document patient medical histories

   D. To classify diseases and conditions

2. HCPCS Level II codes are primarily used for:

   A. Inpatient procedures

   B. Outpatient procedures

   C. Durable medical equipment, prosthetics, orthotics, and supplies

   D. Diagnostic laboratory tests

3. Modifier -25 is used to indicate:

   A. A bilateral procedure

   B. A significant, separately identifiable E/M service by the same physician on the same day of the procedure

   C. Professional component of a service

   D. Technical component of a service

4. Which modifier indicates a bilateral procedure?

   A. -25

   B. -50

C. -26

D. -TC

5. The CPT code for a comprehensive outpatient evaluation and management visit for a new patient could be:

A. 99203

B. 99213

C. 99223

D. 99233

6. A HCPCS Level II code for a knee brace might begin with which letter?

A. A

B. E

C. L

D. J

7. Which of the following scenarios would most likely use a HCPCS Level II code?

A. A complex brain surgery

B. A routine physical examination

C. An influenza vaccination

D. An MRI of the spine

8. Modifier -59 is used to indicate:

  A. A distinct procedural service

  B. An extended service

  C. A repeat procedure by the same physician

  D. Multiple procedures

9. Which of the following is true about modifiers in CPT coding?

  A. They are optional and rarely impact reimbursement

  B. They provide additional information that can affect payment

  C. They are only used for surgical procedures

  D. They replace the need for detailed medical documentation

10. HCPCS codes are updated:

  A. Monthly

  B. Quarterly

  C. Annually

  D. Biennially

Answers

1. B. To report medical, surgical, and diagnostic services for billing

2. C. Durable medical equipment, prosthetics, orthotics, and supplies

3. B. A significant, separately identifiable E/M service by the same physician on the same day of the procedure

4. B. -50

5. A. 99203

6. C. L

7. C. An influenza vaccination

8. A. A distinct procedural service

9. B. They provide additional information that can affect payment

10. C. Annually

These questions and answers are designed to reinforce your understanding of the CPT and HCPCS coding systems, emphasizing the importance of accuracy, specificity, and up-to-date knowledge in medical coding practices.

Chapter 6: Advanced CPT and HCPCS Coding

6.1. CPT Coding for Complex Procedures

Advanced CPT coding for complex procedures involves navigating intricate details and applying specific guidelines to ensure accurate representation of medical services. These procedures may span across various medical specialties and require a deep understanding of coding rules, the use of modifiers, and the ability to interpret comprehensive clinical documentation. Let's delve into the nuances of CPT coding for complex procedures, highlighting key considerations and strategies for accurate coding.

Understanding Complex Procedures

Complex procedures are those that involve multiple steps, extensive use of technology, or high levels of skill and expertise. Examples include certain surgical interventions, advanced diagnostic tests, and sophisticated treatments like robotic surgeries, complex spine surgeries, and multi-component chemotherapy regimens.

Key Considerations for Coding Complex Procedures

- **Comprehensive Documentation:** Detailed documentation is paramount for coding complex procedures. It should clearly describe every aspect of the procedure, including preparatory steps, the procedure itself, and post-operative care.

- **Multiple Codes vs. Single Comprehensive Code:** Some complex procedures may be adequately described by a single, comprehensive CPT code, while others may require multiple codes to capture all components of the procedure. Determining the most appropriate approach depends on the guidelines provided in the CPT manual and any specific instructions for the codes in question.

- **Use of Modifiers:** Modifiers play a critical role in coding complex procedures. They can indicate that a procedure was more extensive than usual, performed on multiple sites, or completed using a special technique. Familiarity with modifiers and their correct application is essential for accurate coding.

- **Global Surgical Package:** Understanding the concept of the global surgical package is crucial when coding for surgical procedures. This package includes pre-operative, intra-operative, and post-operative services related to the surgery. Coders must identify services outside of this package that require separate coding.

Strategies for Coding Complex Procedures

1. **Analyze the Entire Procedure:** Begin by reviewing the entire procedure documentation to understand its scope and components. This holistic view aids in identifying all elements that may require coding.

2. **Refer to the CPT Manual:** Use the CPT manual to find applicable codes, paying close attention to any notes, guidelines, and instructions related to complex procedures.

3. **Identify Primary and Secondary Codes:** Determine the primary procedure code that represents the main aspect of the service provided. Then, identify any additional codes needed to capture secondary or ancillary aspects of the procedure.

4. **Apply Modifiers Appropriately:** Use modifiers to provide additional details about the procedure, such as -22 for procedures that are more complex than usually required or -59 for distinct procedural services.

5. **Stay Informed About Updates:** CPT codes and guidelines for complex procedures can change. Stay updated with annual CPT updates, specialty society guidelines, and payer policies.

6. **Collaborate with Healthcare Providers:** When documentation is unclear or insufficient for accurate coding, collaborate with healthcare providers to clarify details about the procedure.

Conclusion

Coding for complex procedures demands a high level of precision and expertise in CPT coding. By thoroughly understanding procedural documentation, applying relevant codes and modifiers, and staying current with coding updates and guidelines, coders can accurately capture the intricacies of complex medical services. This not only ensures appropriate reimbursement but also contributes to the integrity of medical records and the overall quality of healthcare data.

6.2. Specialized Coding in HCPCS

Healthcare Common Procedure Coding System (HCPCS) Level II codes are an essential part of the medical billing and coding landscape, providing a standardized coding system for services, procedures, and supplies not covered by the Current Procedural Terminology (CPT) codes. Specialized coding in HCPCS involves understanding and applying these codes to accurately represent a wide range of healthcare services and items, including durable medical equipment (DME), prosthetics, orthotics, medications, and other services that are integral to patient care.

Key Aspects of Specialized Coding in HCPCS

1. Durable Medical Equipment (DME):

DME is any equipment that provides therapeutic benefits to a patient in need because of certain medical conditions or illnesses. HCPCS codes in the "E" series are used to bill for items like wheelchairs, hospital beds, and oxygen equipment. Accurate coding requires detailed knowledge of the equipment, including its features and how it's used by the patient.

2. Prosthetics and Orthotics:

Prosthetic devices replace missing body parts, while orthotic devices support or correct the function of a body part. Coding for these items, typically found under the "L" series in HCPCS, demands specificity regarding the item provided, its customization, and any fitting services rendered.

3. Medications and Injections:

Many medications, especially those administered in a clinical setting, are coded using HCPCS Level II, particularly in the "J" series. This includes chemotherapy drugs, vaccines, and injectable medications. Coders must be precise in reporting the drug's name, dosage, and route of administration.

4. Ambulance Services and Transportation:

HCPCS codes also cover non-emergency and emergency transportation services to medical facilities, coded under the "A" series. These codes capture details about the mode of transport, the reason for the transport, and the patient's condition.

5. Supplies and Miscellaneous Services:

From surgical supplies to diagnostic tests not covered under CPT codes, HCPCS Level II codes include a broad category of miscellaneous items and services. Coders must navigate these codes, often found in the "A," "S," and "K" series, to ensure comprehensive billing for patient care services.

Strategies for Effective Specialized Coding in HCPCS

- **Stay Updated:** HCPCS Level II codes are updated annually to reflect changes in healthcare practices and technologies. Staying informed about these updates is critical for maintaining coding accuracy.

- **Understand Documentation Requirements:** Thorough documentation from healthcare providers is essential for justifying the use of certain HCPCS codes, especially for items like DME and prosthetics that require detailed descriptions.

- **Utilize Payer Guidelines:** Since payer policies can vary, understanding the specific requirements and guidelines of different insurers for HCPCS-coded items and services is vital for successful reimbursement.

- **Engage in Continuous Education:** Specialized areas within HCPCS coding often require specific knowledge and expertise. Coders should pursue ongoing education and training opportunities to stay competent in these areas.

Conclusion

Specialized coding in HCPCS Level II plays a pivotal role in the healthcare reimbursement system, covering a diverse range of services and items not included in the CPT coding system. By mastering these codes, healthcare coders ensure that providers are accurately reimbursed for the essential services and supplies they offer to patients, supporting the overall goal of delivering effective and comprehensive healthcare.

6.3. Challenges in CPT and HCPCS Coding

Navigating the complexities of CPT (Current Procedural Terminology) and HCPCS (Healthcare Common Procedure Coding System) coding presents several challenges for medical coders. These challenges stem from the dynamic nature of healthcare services, continuous updates to coding systems, and the intricate details required for accurate coding. Addressing these challenges is essential for ensuring accurate billing, compliance, and efficient healthcare delivery.

1. Keeping Up with Updates

Both CPT and HCPCS codes are updated annually to reflect advancements in medical technology, new procedures, and changes in healthcare practices.

- **Challenge:** Coders must stay informed about these updates to ensure coding practices remain current and compliant.

- **Solution:** Regular participation in professional development courses, webinars, and seminars is crucial. Utilizing resources from the American Medical Association (AMA) for CPT updates and the Centers for Medicare & Medicaid Services (CMS) for HCPCS updates can also be beneficial.

2. Coding for New Technologies and Procedures

As medical science evolves, new technologies and procedures emerge that may not have direct equivalents in existing coding systems.

- **Challenge:** Finding the most appropriate code for innovative procedures or technologies can be difficult, particularly when specific codes have not yet been established.

- **Solution:** Coders should leverage Category III CPT codes designed for emerging technologies and consult payer policies for guidance on coding novel procedures.

3. Documentation Quality and Specificity

Accurate coding depends heavily on the quality and specificity of clinical documentation provided by healthcare providers.

- **Challenge:** Incomplete or nonspecific documentation can lead to coding inaccuracies, claim denials, and underpayment.

- **Solution:** Coders should work closely with healthcare providers to improve documentation practices, emphasizing the importance of detailed and specific clinical information. Implementing regular documentation training for providers can also help.

4. Correct Use of Modifiers

Modifiers in CPT and HCPCS coding add specificity to services provided but can complicate the coding process.

- **Challenge:** Incorrect application of modifiers can lead to reimbursement issues and compliance risks.

- **Solution:** Coders need thorough knowledge of modifier rules and should review each case carefully to determine the necessity and accuracy of modifier use. Regular auditing of modifier usage can also identify and correct common errors.

5. Navigating Payer-Specific Policies

Insurance payers may have unique guidelines for how certain codes should be applied, which can differ from standard coding practices.

- **Challenge:** Coders must navigate these variations to ensure claims are compliant with each payer's policies, which can vary widely and change frequently.

- **Solution:** Establishing a database of payer-specific guidelines and maintaining open communication with insurance representatives can help coders stay informed about policy changes. Additionally, attending payer-specific training sessions can provide valuable insights.

6. Specialized Coding Requirements

Some areas of healthcare require highly specialized coding knowledge, such as coding for oncology, cardiology, or behavioral health.

- **Challenge:** Coders may struggle with the intricacies of coding in specialized fields without additional training or resources.

- **Solution:** Investing in specialized training or certification in areas of high need within the coding team can enhance accuracy and efficiency. Collaboration with clinical specialists to understand complex services can also improve coding outcomes.

Conclusion

CPT and HCPCS coding are critical components of the healthcare reimbursement system, requiring coders to navigate a landscape marked by continuous change and complexity. Addressing the challenges in coding requires a commitment to ongoing education, collaboration with healthcare providers, and strategic use of resources and tools. By overcoming these challenges, coders play a vital role in supporting accurate billing, compliance, and the financial sustainability of healthcare organizations.

6.4. Keeping Up with CPT and HCPCS Updates

Staying current with updates to the CPT (Current Procedural Terminology) and HCPCS (Healthcare Common Procedure Coding System) codes is crucial for medical coders, billing professionals, and healthcare providers. These updates can significantly impact billing, reimbursement, and compliance processes. Here are strategies and resources to effectively manage and stay informed about these critical updates.

Understanding the Importance of Updates

1. **Reflects New Procedures and Technologies:** Updates incorporate new medical procedures and technologies, ensuring coding reflects current medical practice.

2. **Adjusts to Regulatory Changes:** Changes may respond to regulatory requirements, affecting how services are billed and reimbursed.

3. **Corrects or Clarifies Existing Codes:** Updates can also correct errors or clarify the use of existing codes to improve coding accuracy and reduce billing errors.

Strategies for Staying Updated

1. Utilize Official Resources:

- **CPT Updates:** The American Medical Association (AMA) releases annual updates to the CPT codes. Their website and publications, such as the AMA CPT® Professional Edition, are authoritative resources for learning about new, revised, and deleted codes.

- **HCPCS Updates:** The Centers for Medicare & Medicaid Services (CMS) manage HCPCS updates, which are typically released annually. The CMS website provides detailed information on HCPCS Level II code changes, including additions, deletions, and modifications.

2. Subscribe to Industry Publications and Newsletters:

- Many professional associations and industry groups publish newsletters and journals that highlight significant coding updates and provide expert commentary on their application.

3. Participate in Professional Development and Training:

- Engage in ongoing education through workshops, webinars, and conferences that focus on coding updates. These events often provide insights into the practical application of new codes and changes to coding guidelines.

4. Leverage Coding Software and Tools:

- Ensure that electronic health records (EHR) systems and coding software are updated to reflect the latest codes. Many software providers also include features that alert users to changes and provide educational resources.

5. Join Professional Associations:

- Membership in professional associations, such as the American Academy of Professional Coders (AAPC) or the American Health Information Management Association (AHIMA), offers access to a wealth of resources, including coding updates, forums, and networking opportunities with peers who can share insights and advice.

6. Collaborate with Peers:

- Engage in discussions with colleagues and participate in online forums where coders share experiences, challenges, and strategies for adapting to coding updates.

Challenges and Solutions

- **Challenge:** Keeping up with the volume of changes can be overwhelming.

  - **Solution:** Focus on changes most relevant to your practice or specialization first. Utilize summary resources and targeted training to manage the workload.

- **Challenge:** Applying new codes correctly requires understanding their context and guidelines.

  - **Solution:** Supplement code updates with practical examples and case studies. Seek clarification from coding experts and professional associations when needed.

Conclusion

Staying current with CPT and HCPCS updates is a continuous process that demands proactive engagement and utilization of various resources. By implementing effective strategies for learning and applying these updates, coding professionals can ensure accuracy in coding practices, optimize reimbursement, and maintain compliance with evolving healthcare standards. This proactive approach ultimately supports the delivery of high-quality healthcare services.

6.5. Exercise: 10 MCQs with Answers at the End

Test your knowledge on advanced CPT and HCPCS coding, including complex procedures, specialized coding, coding challenges, and updates. Answers are provided at the end for self-assessment.

Questions

1. What is the primary purpose of annual updates to CPT and HCPCS codes?

   A. To complicate the coding process

   B. To reflect changes in medical technology and practices

   C. To reduce the number of available codes

D. To increase healthcare costs

2. Which resource is essential for finding authoritative updates on CPT coding?

A. World Health Organization (WHO)

B. American Medical Association (AMA)

C. Centers for Disease Control and Prevention (CDC)

D. National Institutes of Health (NIH)

3. A comprehensive update to HCPCS codes is managed by:

A. AMA

B. WHO

C. CMS

D. FDA

4. Modifier -22 is used to indicate:

A. A bilateral procedure

B. An increased procedural service

C. A service performed multiple times

D. A technical component

5. For coding a complex spine surgery involving multiple levels, a coder might need to:

A. Use a single comprehensive code

B. Apply multiple codes to represent each level addressed

C. Use an unspecified procedure code

D. Omit coding for the complexity to simplify the process

6. HCPCS Level II codes for Durable Medical Equipment (DME) start with which letter?

A. A

B. D

C. E

D. M

7. The use of a -59 modifier indicates:

A. A distinct procedural service

B. Professional component

C. Bilateral procedure

D. Reduced services

8. Specialized coding in HCPCS often requires knowledge of:

A. Only outpatient procedures

B. Diagnostic tests and laboratory services

C. Drugs, supplies, and DME

D. Inpatient surgical procedures only

9. Continuous education and staying informed about coding updates can be achieved through:

A. Attending only the mandatory training sessions

B. Relying solely on software updates for information

C. Participating in workshops, webinars, and professional associations

D. Ignoring updates until they are several years old

10. A primary challenge in coding with the latest CPT and HCPCS updates includes:

A. Finding codes that have been deliberately hidden

B. Applying new codes without understanding their implications

C. Memorizing the entire code set annually

D. Using outdated codes deliberately for simplicity

Answers

1. B. To reflect changes in medical technology and practices

2. B. American Medical Association (AMA)

3. C. CMS

4. B. An increased procedural service

5. B. Apply multiple codes to represent each level addressed

6. C. E

7. A. A distinct procedural service

8. C. Drugs, supplies, and DME

9. C. Participating in workshops, webinars, and professional associations

10. B. Applying new codes without understanding their implications

These questions highlight the importance of staying current with CPT and HCPCS coding updates, understanding the use of modifiers, and the challenges faced in accurately coding complex procedures and specialized areas.

Chapter 7: Introduction to Billing and Reimbursement

7.1. Basics of Medical Billing

Medical billing is a critical component of the healthcare revenue cycle, bridging the gap between healthcare service delivery and payment. It involves the preparation and submission of claims to insurance companies and payers to receive payment for services provided by healthcare professionals. Understanding the basics of medical billing is essential for ensuring that healthcare facilities are compensated accurately and promptly for the services they render.

Key Components of Medical Billing

1. Patient Registration and Verification:

The billing process begins at the patient's first point of contact, where personal and insurance information is collected and verified. Accurate patient information is crucial for ensuring claims are submitted to the correct payer.

2. Coding of Services:

Medical coding translates healthcare services, procedures, and diagnoses into standardized codes. CPT, HCPCS, and ICD-10 codes are used to accurately describe the services provided, which is essential for billing and reimbursement.

3. Charge Capture and Entry:

This step involves recording all chargeable services provided to the patient. It's vital to capture every service accurately to ensure complete billing for all care delivered.

4. Claim Submission:

Claims are prepared and submitted to insurance companies electronically or via paper forms. The claim includes detailed information about the patient, provider, services provided, and the codes that describe those services.

5. Payment Posting:

Once a claim is processed by the payer, payment is sent to the healthcare provider. Payment posting involves recording these payments, adjustments, and any patient responsibilities in the billing system.

6. Patient Billing:

After insurance payments are applied, any remaining balance is billed to the patient. This may include deductibles, copayments, and services not covered by insurance.

7. Follow-Up and Appeals:

Claims may be denied or underpaid by insurance companies for various reasons. Follow-up includes managing denials, submitting additional information if needed, and appealing decisions when appropriate.

Challenges in Medical Billing

- **Denials and Rejections:** Claims may be denied due to errors, incomplete information, or non-covered services. Managing these issues requires thorough review and timely resubmission or appeal.

- **Changing Payer Policies:** Insurance companies frequently update their policies and coverage guidelines, necessitating ongoing education and adaptation by billing staff.

- **Patient Financial Responsibility:** With the rise of high-deductible health plans, collecting payments from patients can be challenging. Clear communication about financial responsibilities is essential.

Strategies for Effective Medical Billing

- **Invest in Training:** Regular training for billing staff on coding updates, payer policies, and billing best practices is essential for minimizing errors and denials.

- **Utilize Technology:** Electronic health records (EHR) and billing software can streamline the billing process, reduce errors, and expedite claim submission and follow-up.

- **Clear Communication:** Providing patients with clear information about their financial responsibilities and the billing process can improve patient satisfaction and reduce collection issues.

Conclusion

Medical billing is a complex but vital process that ensures healthcare providers are reimbursed for the services they deliver. By understanding the fundamentals of medical billing, healthcare organizations can navigate the challenges of reimbursement, maintain financial health, and continue to provide quality care to their patients. Effective medical billing requires accuracy, attention to detail, and a commitment to continuous improvement and adaptation to the ever-changing healthcare landscape.

7.2. The Reimbursement Process

The reimbursement process in healthcare is a critical pathway through which healthcare providers receive payment for their services from insurance companies or directly from patients. This process involves several steps, each essential for ensuring that providers are compensated accurately and in a timely manner for the care they deliver. Understanding this process is fundamental for managing the financial operations of healthcare facilities and for ensuring access to healthcare services for patients.

Steps in the Reimbursement Process

1. Service Delivery:

The process begins with the provision of healthcare services to the patient. Detailed records of the services provided, including diagnoses, procedures, and treatments, are essential for accurate billing.

2. Medical Coding:

After services are delivered, medical coders translate the details of the patient's visit into standardized codes using ICD-10 for diagnoses, CPT for procedures and services, and HCPCS for other services and supplies. Accurate coding is critical for describing the care provided in a universally recognized language.

**3. Charge Capture and Claim Preparation:

Charge capture involves documenting all the chargeable services provided to a patient. These charges are then compiled into a claim, which details the patient's information, services provided, and the corresponding codes.

4. Claim Submission:

The prepared claim is submitted to the insurance company or payer. Claims can be submitted electronically, which is faster and allows for easier tracking, or via paper forms in some cases.

5. Claim Review and Adjudication:

Upon receiving the claim, the payer reviews it to verify its accuracy and compliance with billing rules and the patient's insurance policy. The adjudication process determines the payer's responsibility and how much will be paid to the provider.

6. Payment and Remittance Advice:

After adjudication, the payer issues payment to the healthcare provider, typically through electronic funds transfer or a check. Along with the payment, the payer sends a remittance advice, detailing how the payment was determined, including any deductions or denials.

7. Balance Billing:

If there is a remaining balance not covered by insurance, such as copayments, deductibles, or non-covered services, the healthcare provider will bill the patient directly for these amounts.

8. Denials and Appeals:

Claims may be denied for various reasons, including errors in coding, lack of medical necessity, or coverage exclusions. Providers can appeal denied claims by submitting additional documentation or correcting errors and resubmitting the claim.

Challenges in the Reimbursement Process

- **Complex Payer Policies:** Navigating the diverse and complex policies of different insurance payers can be challenging, requiring constant updates and training.

- **Coding Errors:** Errors in medical coding can lead to claim denials or underpayments, necessitating meticulous review and correction processes.

- **Delays in Payment:** Delays in the adjudication process or in issuing payment can impact the financial operations of healthcare providers.

Strategies for Optimizing the Reimbursement Process

- **Invest in Education and Training:** Regular training for coding and billing staff on the latest coding standards and payer policies is essential.

- **Leverage Technology:** Utilizing advanced billing software and electronic health records can streamline the billing process, reduce errors, and expedite payments.

- **Effective Communication:** Clear communication with patients about their financial responsibilities and with insurance companies during the adjudication process can reduce delays and improve the efficiency of the reimbursement process.

Conclusion

The reimbursement process is a cornerstone of the healthcare system, ensuring that providers are compensated for their services and that patients have access to necessary care. By understanding and effectively managing this process, healthcare providers can maintain financial stability, support patient care, and navigate the complexities of healthcare billing and insurance.

7.3. Understanding Insurance Plans and Payer Requirements

Navigating the landscape of insurance plans and payer requirements is crucial for healthcare providers to ensure accurate billing and maximize reimbursement. Insurance plans can vary significantly in terms of coverage, patient responsibility, and the processes for claim submission and payment. Understanding these differences is key to effective healthcare management and patient care coordination.

Types of Insurance Plans

1. Private Health Insurance:

- **Preferred Provider Organizations (PPOs):** Offer patients more flexibility in choosing healthcare providers and do not require referrals for specialists. Out-of-network care is available but at a higher cost to the patient.

- **Health Maintenance Organizations (HMOs):** Require patients to choose a primary care physician (PCP) who coordinates all care and provides referrals for specialists. Typically, only in-network providers are covered.

- **Exclusive Provider Organizations (EPOs):** Similar to PPOs but without coverage for out-of-network care, except in emergencies.

- **High Deductible Health Plans (HDHPs):** Feature higher deductibles and lower premiums, often combined with Health Savings Accounts (HSAs) allowing patients to save money tax-free for medical expenses.

2. Government Insurance Programs:

- **Medicare:** A federal program for people aged 65 and older, and for some younger individuals with disabilities or specific conditions. It includes Part A (hospital insurance), Part B (medical insurance), Part C (Medicare Advantage Plans), and Part D (prescription drug coverage).

- **Medicaid:** A joint federal and state program that provides health coverage to eligible low-income adults, children, pregnant women, elderly adults, and people with disabilities.

- **Children's Health Insurance Program (CHIP):** Provides coverage to eligible children, through both Medicaid and separate CHIP programs.

Understanding Payer Requirements

Each insurance payer has specific requirements regarding claim submission, documentation, pre-authorizations, and appeals. Familiarity with these requirements is essential for compliance and to minimize claim denials or delays.

Key Aspects Include:

- **Pre-Authorization and Referrals:** Some services or medications may require prior authorization from the insurance company, or a referral from a PCP in the case of HMO plans.

- **Timely Filing Limits:** Insurance payers have specific deadlines for submitting claims and appealing denials, which must be adhered to for successful reimbursement.

- **Documentation Standards:** Payers require detailed and specific documentation to support the medical necessity of services billed.

- **Coding Guidelines:** Accurate use of ICD-10, CPT, and HCPCS codes according to payer-specific guidelines is crucial for claim acceptance.

Strategies for Managing Insurance Requirements

- **Stay Informed:** Regularly review payer contracts, bulletins, and updates to stay informed about changes in policies and requirements.

- **Effective Communication:** Establish clear lines of communication with insurance representatives to resolve issues and clarify policies.

- **Patient Education:** Inform patients about their insurance benefits, coverage limits, and financial responsibilities to reduce confusion and ensure timely payment.

- **Utilize Technology:** Leverage electronic health record (EHR) systems and billing software that can help manage payer requirements, track claim statuses, and flag potential issues before claim submission.

Conclusion

Understanding the diverse landscape of insurance plans and payer requirements is integral to the financial health of healthcare practices and the provision of patient care. By adopting strategies to stay informed and effectively manage these requirements, healthcare providers can streamline the billing process, reduce claim denials, and enhance patient satisfaction with the financial aspects of their care.

7.4. Billing for Various Healthcare Settings

Billing practices in healthcare vary significantly across different settings, each with its unique challenges and requirements. From hospitals and outpatient clinics to telehealth services and home health care, understanding the nuances of billing for each setting is crucial for accurate reimbursement and compliance. Let's explore the billing considerations for various healthcare settings.

1. Hospital Inpatient Billing

- **Complexity:** Hospital inpatient billing involves charges for room and board, medications, treatments, procedures, and any other care provided during the stay.

- **DRG System:** Reimbursement is often based on Diagnosis-Related Groups (DRG), which categorize hospitalization costs for particular conditions or procedures, incentivizing efficient care delivery.

- **Key Consideration:** Accurate documentation and coding of diagnoses and procedures are crucial to determine the correct DRG and ensure appropriate reimbursement.

2. Outpatient and Ambulatory Care

- **Services Covered:** Includes services provided in outpatient departments, ambulatory surgical centers, and clinics, ranging from diagnostic tests to minor surgical procedures.

- **Billing Process:** Billing is typically based on the specific services provided, using CPT codes to describe each service, procedure, or test performed.

- **Key Consideration:** Outpatient billing must carefully distinguish between facility fees and professional fees for services rendered, as they are billed separately.

3. Telehealth Services

- **Growth and Acceptance:** The use of telehealth has expanded rapidly, offering remote consultations, evaluations, and some treatments.

- **Billing Guidelines:** Specific CPT and HCPCS codes have been developed or designated for telehealth services, with payers providing guidelines for their use.

- **Key Consideration:** Providers must stay informed about evolving payer policies regarding telehealth, especially as emergency measures introduced during public health emergencies may change.

4. Home Health Care

- **Services Offered:** Home health care encompasses a wide range of healthcare services delivered at a patient's home, from nursing care to physical therapy.

- **Reimbursement Models:** Billing for home health care often involves per-visit rates or episodic payment models, depending on the payer and services provided.

- **Key Consideration:** Documentation of medical necessity and adherence to plan of care are vital for billing and compliance in home health care settings.

5. Long-Term Care and Rehabilitation Facilities

- **Scope of Care:** These facilities provide long-term nursing care, rehabilitation services, and assistance with daily living activities for patients with chronic conditions or recovering from illness or injury.

- **Billing Considerations:** Billing may involve daily rates for custodial care, along with charges for additional medical or therapeutic services provided.

- **Key Consideration:** Understanding payer-specific guidelines for long-term care coverage, including Medicare and Medicaid limitations, is essential.

Strategies for Effective Billing Across Settings

- **Comprehensive Training:** Ensure billing staff are trained in the specific requirements and nuances of billing for different healthcare settings.

- **Stay Updated:** Keep abreast of changes in billing regulations, payer policies, and coding updates relevant to each setting.

- **Leverage Technology:** Utilize advanced billing software and electronic health records (EHR) systems that can accommodate the diverse billing needs of various healthcare settings.

- **Audit and Compliance:** Regularly review billing practices through audits to ensure accuracy and compliance, minimizing the risk of errors and denials.

Conclusion

Billing in diverse healthcare settings requires a nuanced understanding of each setting's specific services, reimbursement models, and regulatory requirements. By adopting setting-specific strategies and maintaining a commitment to continuous learning and compliance, healthcare providers can navigate the complexities of billing across different care environments, ensuring financial stability and the continued provision of high-quality care.

7.5. Exercise: 10 MCQs with Answers at the End

Test your knowledge on the introduction to billing and reimbursement, including the basics of medical billing, the reimbursement process, understanding insurance plans and payer requirements, and billing for various healthcare settings. Answers are provided at the end for self-assessment.

Questions

1. What is the first step in the medical billing process?

    A. Claim Submission

    B. Service Delivery

    C. Payment Posting

    D. Patient Registration and Verification

2. DRGs are primarily used in billing for which type of care?

    A. Outpatient care

    B. Inpatient hospital stays

    C. Telehealth services

    D. Home health care

3. Which coding system is used to code diagnoses on claims for all types of care?

    A. CPT

    B. HCPCS Level II

    C. ICD-10-CM

    D. DRG

4. What does a -25 modifier indicate when attached to a CPT code?

A. Bilateral procedure

B. Significant, separately identifiable E/M service

C. Professional component

D. Technical component

5. Medicare is a healthcare program for:

A. Children under 18

B. Low-income families

C. Individuals aged 65 and older or with certain disabilities

D. Veterans and military personnel

6. Which setting typically uses a per-visit rate or episodic payment model for billing?

A. Telehealth services

B. Hospital inpatient care

C. Home health care

D. Outpatient clinics

7. A key consideration for billing telehealth services is:

    A. Determining the patient's income level

    B. Staying informed about evolving payer policies

    C. Always using in-person visit codes for billing

    D. Sending a physical bill to the patient's home address

8. For outpatient and ambulatory care billing, it's important to distinguish between:

    A. Facility fees and professional fees

    B. DRGs and ICD-10-CM codes

    C. Inpatient and outpatient DRGs

    D. E/M codes and procedure codes

9. In the reimbursement process, what is the term for the detailed explanation of how a payment was determined by the payer?

    A. Claim

    B. Invoice

    C. Remittance Advice

    D. EOB (Explanation of Benefits)

10. Prior authorization is most likely required for:

A. Routine physical examinations

B. Emergency room visits

C. Certain medications or procedures specified by the insurance plan

D. All outpatient visits

Answers

1. D. Patient Registration and Verification

2. B. Inpatient hospital stays

3. C. ICD-10-CM

4. B. Significant, separately identifiable E/M service

5. C. Individuals aged 65 and older or with certain disabilities

6. C. Home health care

7. B. Staying informed about evolving payer policies

8. A. Facility fees and professional fees

9. C. Remittance Advice

10. C. Certain medications or procedures specified by the insurance plan

These questions and answers are designed to reinforce your understanding of key concepts in medical billing and reimbursement, highlighting the importance of accurate coding, understanding insurance plans, and navigating billing for different healthcare settings.

Chapter 8: Advanced Billing Techniques

8.1. Navigating Complex Billing Scenarios

Advanced billing techniques are essential for managing complex billing scenarios that arise in healthcare settings. These scenarios often involve unique patient situations, intricate insurance plan stipulations, or specific regulatory requirements that necessitate a deep understanding of billing practices and payer policies. Successfully navigating these scenarios ensures that healthcare providers are reimbursed accurately for the services they provide, while also maintaining compliance with healthcare laws and regulations.

Identifying Complex Billing Scenarios

Complex billing scenarios can include:

- **Multiple Insurers:** Patients covered by more than one insurance plan, requiring coordination of benefits to determine primary and secondary payers.

- **Out-of-Network Services:** Services provided by clinicians or facilities not within a patient's insurance network, affecting reimbursement rates and out-of-pocket costs.

- **High-cost Treatments and Procedures:** Specialized treatments, such as certain surgeries or chemotherapy, may have specific billing requirements and need prior authorization.

- **Bundled Payments and Case Rates:** Some services are reimbursed as a single bundled payment rather than individually, requiring accurate coding to capture the entire episode of care.

Strategies for Navigating Complex Billing Scenarios

1. Thorough Verification of Benefits:

- Conduct detailed insurance verifications for each patient visit to understand coverage limits, deductibles, copayments, and prior authorization requirements.

2. Coordination of Benefits (COB):

- For patients with multiple insurance plans, determine the order of responsibility to ensure claims are submitted correctly to the primary and secondary insurers.

3. Understanding and Applying Payer Policies:

- Stay updated on individual payer policies, especially for out-of-network benefits and procedures that require prior authorization.

4. Accurate Coding and Use of Modifiers:

- Utilize the correct codes and modifiers to describe complex treatments accurately. This includes understanding bundled payments and how to code for multiple procedures.

5. Clear Patient Communication:

- Inform patients about their financial responsibilities, especially for out-of-network services or treatments that may not be fully covered by insurance.

6. Regular Training and Education:

- Engage in continuous education on advanced billing practices, payer policies, and regulatory changes to stay competent in managing complex billing scenarios.

Challenges in Complex Billing Scenarios

- **Denials and Delays:** Incorrect billing in complex scenarios often leads to claim denials or payment delays, impacting cash flow.

- **Compliance Risks:** Failing to adhere to payer policies and healthcare regulations can result in compliance issues and financial penalties.

- **Patient Dissatisfaction:** Miscommunication or misunderstandings about billing can lead to patient dissatisfaction and disputes.

Solutions for Effective Management

- **Utilize Advanced Billing Software:** Employ billing software that can handle complex billing scenarios, including the management of COB and the application of payer-specific rules.

- **Implement Quality Assurance Processes:** Regular audits and checks can identify and rectify billing errors before claim submission.

- **Develop a Dedicated Team:** Consider having a team specialized in handling complex billing scenarios, equipped with the expertise to navigate the intricacies of advanced billing techniques.

Conclusion

Navigating complex billing scenarios requires a multifaceted approach that combines in-depth knowledge of billing practices, payer policies, and regulatory requirements. By implementing strategic measures, healthcare providers can effectively manage these scenarios, ensuring accurate billing, timely reimbursement, and sustained compliance. Continuous education and the use of technology play vital roles in mastering advanced billing techniques and overcoming the challenges presented by complex billing scenarios.

8.2. Billing for High-Risk or Specialized Procedures

Billing for high-risk or specialized procedures presents unique challenges due to the complexity of the services provided, the level of expertise required, and the potential for higher costs. These procedures often demand precise coding, thorough documentation, and a deep understanding of payer policies to ensure accurate reimbursement. Here's a guide on how to navigate the billing intricacies for these critical healthcare services.

Understanding High-Risk or Specialized Procedures

High-risk or specialized procedures can include advanced surgical operations, innovative treatments for rare conditions, or complex diagnostic tests. Examples include organ transplants, certain cancer therapies like CAR-T cell therapy, and advanced neurosurgery. The high cost, advanced technology, and specialized care associated with these procedures necessitate a detailed billing approach.

Key Billing Considerations

1. Precise Coding:

- Accurate coding is paramount, often requiring the use of specific CPT and HCPCS codes that reflect the complexity and specificity of the procedure. Modifiers may also be necessary to indicate specific circumstances of the care provided.

2. Detailed Documentation:

- Comprehensive documentation must support the medical necessity of the procedure, detailing the patient's condition, the rationale for choosing the specific treatment, and the expected outcomes. This documentation is critical for justifying the procedure to payers.

3. Prior Authorization:

- Many high-risk or specialized procedures require prior authorization from the payer to confirm that the procedure is covered under the patient's plan and is medically necessary. Obtaining prior authorization is a crucial step to avoid denials.

4. Coordination with Multiple Departments:

- Billing for these procedures often involves coordination between multiple departments within a healthcare facility, including the surgical team, the billing department, and case management, to ensure all aspects of the procedure are accurately captured and billed.

5. Understanding Payer Policies:

- Familiarity with the specific policies of various payers regarding specialized procedures is essential. Policies may vary significantly regarding coverage, reimbursement rates, and required documentation.

Strategies for Effective Billing

1. Engage in Continuous Education:

- Stay updated on coding changes, payer policies, and advancements in medical procedures to ensure billing practices remain current.

2. Leverage Expertise:

- Consider consulting with or employing billing specialists who have experience in high-risk or specialized procedures to navigate the complexities effectively.

3. Utilize Advanced Billing Software:

- Implement billing software that can accommodate the detailed coding and documentation requirements of specialized procedures.

4. Communicate with Payers:

- Establish open lines of communication with insurance payers to clarify coverage details, discuss prior authorization requirements, and resolve any disputes or denials promptly.

5. Educate Patients:

- Inform patients about the billing process for specialized procedures, including potential costs, insurance coverage, and the possibility of financial assistance programs.

Challenges and Solutions

- **Challenge:** Managing the extensive documentation and justification required for high-risk procedures.

- **Solution:** Implement a systematic approach to documentation that includes checklists and templates to ensure all necessary information is captured.

- **Challenge:** Navigating payer denials or underpayments for complex procedures.

- **Solution:** Develop a robust appeals process, backed by detailed documentation and a clear understanding of payer policies.

Conclusion

Billing for high-risk or specialized procedures requires a comprehensive approach that encompasses accurate coding, detailed documentation, and thorough knowledge of payer policies. By adopting targeted strategies and leveraging expertise, healthcare providers can navigate the challenges associated with these procedures, ensuring appropriate reimbursement and supporting the delivery of advanced medical care.

8.3. Appeals and Denials Management

In the realm of medical billing, handling appeals and managing denials are critical aspects that can significantly impact a healthcare provider's revenue cycle. An appeal is a formal request to reconsider a denial or underpayment, while a denial is a refusal by an insurance company to honor a request for payment. Understanding how to effectively manage these scenarios is crucial for recovering rightfully owed revenue and ensuring financial stability for healthcare providers.

Understanding Appeals and Denials

Denials can occur for various reasons, including coding errors, lack of medical necessity, failure to obtain prior authorization, and patient eligibility issues. **Appeals** are the next step to contest these denials, requiring a detailed review of the claim, gathering of supporting documentation, and adherence to specific payer guidelines for the appeal process.

Strategies for Effective Appeals and Denials Management

1. Analyze and Categorize Denials:

- Understand the root causes of denials by categorizing them (e.g., coding errors, documentation issues). This helps in developing targeted strategies for prevention and appeal.

2. Develop a Systematic Appeal Process:

- Establish a standardized process for appealing denials, including timelines, documentation requirements, and follow-up procedures. Ensure the team is trained on this process.

3. Timely Response:

- Act promptly to appeal denials, keeping in mind the time limits set by payers. Delayed responses can result in the forfeiture of the right to appeal.

4. Gather Comprehensive Documentation:

- Compile all relevant documentation to support the appeal, including medical records, prior authorizations, and correspondence with the payer. Detailed documentation strengthens the case for reimbursement.

5. Utilize Clear and Concise Communication:

- Appeals should be clear, well-organized, and concise, directly addressing the reasons for denial and providing evidence to counteract these reasons.

6. Monitor and Track Appeals:

- Keep detailed records of all appeals, including submission dates, follow-up actions, and outcomes. This helps in identifying trends and areas for improvement.

7. Engage with Payers:

- Maintain open lines of communication with payers. Understanding their perspective can provide insights into the denial reasons and how to prevent future issues.

8. Continuous Education and Training:

- Keep the billing team updated on coding changes, payer policies, and best practices in appeals management through regular training and education.

Common Challenges in Appeals and Denials Management

- **Complex Payer Policies:** Navigating the varied and complex policies of different insurance payers can be challenging.

- **Resource Intensive:** The appeals process can be time-consuming and resource-intensive, requiring dedicated staff.

- **Maintaining Compliance:** Ensuring that appeals adhere to all regulatory and payer-specific guidelines is crucial for compliance.

Solutions

- **Leverage Technology:** Use billing software and other technologies to streamline the appeals process, track denials, and maintain documentation.

- **Outsource Appeals Management:** Consider outsourcing to companies specializing in appeals and denials management to leverage their expertise and resources.

- **Payer Collaboration:** Work collaboratively with payers to understand their requirements and reduce the likelihood of future denials.

Conclusion

Effective appeals and denials management is essential for maximizing reimbursement and maintaining a healthy revenue cycle in healthcare settings. By understanding the reasons behind denials, developing a systematic approach to appeals, and leveraging resources efficiently, healthcare providers can improve their chances of overturning denials and securing payment for services rendered. Continuous improvement in processes and communication with payers can also help in reducing the incidence of denials over time.

8.4. Billing Compliance and Audits

Billing compliance and audits are critical components of healthcare management, ensuring that billing practices adhere to legal and regulatory requirements. Compliance programs are designed to prevent, detect, and resolve billing errors and fraudulent practices, thereby protecting healthcare providers from legal issues and financial penalties. Audits, both internal and external, are essential tools for assessing the accuracy and integrity of billing processes.

Importance of Billing Compliance

- **Prevents Fraud and Abuse:** Establishes safeguards against billing for services not rendered, upcoding, and other fraudulent practices.

- **Ensures Accurate Billing:** Promotes accurate coding and billing for services provided, ensuring that healthcare providers are reimbursed correctly.

- **Minimizes Legal Risks:** Reduces the risk of penalties, fines, and legal action associated with non-compliance with healthcare billing regulations.

- **Maintains Reputation:** Protects the reputation of healthcare providers by demonstrating a commitment to ethical billing practices.

Components of a Compliance Program

1. **Policies and Procedures:** Develop and implement clear billing and coding policies and procedures that comply with regulatory standards.

2. **Training and Education:** Provide ongoing training for staff on billing procedures, coding standards, and compliance requirements.

3. **Monitoring and Auditing:** Conduct regular internal audits to assess compliance and identify areas for improvement.

4. **Reporting Mechanisms:** Establish confidential channels for staff to report billing inaccuracies or unethical practices without fear of retaliation.

5. **Response and Corrective Action:** Implement processes to investigate reported issues, take corrective action, and prevent future occurrences.

Conducting Billing Audits

Internal Audits:

- Conducted by the healthcare provider to self-assess compliance and accuracy in billing practices. It involves reviewing a sample of claims to identify errors or inconsistencies.

External Audits:

- Performed by outside entities, such as government agencies (e.g., CMS for Medicare and Medicaid audits) or private insurance companies. External audits verify compliance with billing regulations and payer contract terms.

Audit Focus Areas

- **Accuracy of Coded Data:** Verifies that codes used for diagnoses, procedures, and services accurately reflect the patient's medical record.

- **Compliance with Payer Policies:** Ensures that billing practices adhere to the specific requirements of each payer, including prior authorizations and documentation standards.

- **Identification of Fraudulent Practices:** Detects patterns that may indicate fraudulent billing, such as billing for services not provided.

Strategies for Enhancing Billing Compliance

- **Regular Review of Regulations:** Stay updated on changes in billing regulations, coding standards, and payer policies.

- **Invest in Compliance Resources:** Allocate resources for compliance activities, including technology tools, staff training, and hiring compliance specialists.

- **Foster a Culture of Compliance:** Encourage an organizational culture that prioritizes ethical billing practices and compliance through leadership support and staff engagement.

Challenges and Solutions

- **Keeping Up with Regulatory Changes:** The complexity and frequency of changes in healthcare regulations can be challenging.

 - **Solution:** Utilize regulatory alerts and subscribe to professional associations for updates.

- **Resource Constraints:** Limited resources may hinder the implementation of effective compliance programs.

- **Solution:** Prioritize compliance activities that have the highest impact on reducing risk and allocate resources accordingly.

Conclusion

Billing compliance and audits are vital for maintaining the integrity of healthcare billing processes, ensuring accurate reimbursement, and minimizing legal and financial risks. By implementing robust compliance programs, conducting regular audits, and fostering a culture of ethical billing practices, healthcare providers can navigate the complexities of billing compliance and enhance the overall quality of healthcare delivery.

8.5. Exercise: 10 MCQs with Answers at the End

Test your understanding of advanced billing techniques, including navigating complex billing scenarios, billing for high-risk or specialized procedures, appeals and denials management, and billing compliance and audits. Answers are provided at the end for self-assessment.

Questions

1. What is the primary goal of a healthcare billing compliance program?

   A. To increase the organization's revenue

   B. To ensure billing practices adhere to legal and regulatory requirements

   C. To simplify the billing process

   D. To eliminate the need for external audits

2. Which of the following is a common reason for claim denials in healthcare billing?

   A. Using the most recent ICD-10-CM codes

   B. Submitting claims electronically

   C. Lack of medical necessity documentation

   D. Providing patient care

3. Prior authorization is mainly required for:

   A. All outpatient visits

   B. Emergency procedures

   C. High-cost treatments and specialized procedures

   D. Routine wellness checks

4. In billing for high-risk or specialized procedures, what is crucial for justifying the procedure to payers?

   A. The number of procedures performed in the past month

B. Comprehensive documentation

C. The patient's ability to pay

D. The healthcare provider's preference

5. An internal audit in healthcare billing is conducted to:

A. Penalize the billing staff for mistakes

B. Assess the accuracy and compliance of billing practices

C. Increase the workload of the healthcare provider

D. Avoid external audits at all costs

6. Which modifier indicates a significant, separately identifiable evaluation and management service by the same physician on the same day of the procedure?

A. -22

B. -25

C. -50

D. -59

7. Coordination of benefits is essential when:

A. A patient has only one insurance plan

B. A patient is covered by more than one insurance plan

C. The healthcare provider is out-of-network

D. Billing for telehealth services

8. A key component of managing appeals and denials is:

A. Ignoring payer feedback

B. Delaying the submission of appeal documents

C. Analyzing and categorizing denials to understand their root causes

D. Automatically resubmitting denied claims without review

9. Which of the following is an effective strategy for enhancing billing compliance?

A. Minimizing staff training on new billing regulations

B. Regular review of regulations and payer policies

C. Discouraging staff from reporting billing inaccuracies

D. Relying solely on external audits for compliance feedback

10. Billing for telehealth services requires:

A. The same codes as in-person services without modifications

B. Specialized codes or modifiers to specify that the service was delivered remotely

C. Prior authorization for each telehealth session

D. Billing only the patient directly, regardless of insurance coverage

Answers

1. B. To ensure billing practices adhere to legal and regulatory requirements

2. C. Lack of medical necessity documentation

3. C. High-cost treatments and specialized procedures

4. B. Comprehensive documentation

5. B. Assess the accuracy and compliance of billing practices

6. B. -25

7. B. A patient is covered by more than one insurance plan

8. C. Analyzing and categorizing denials to understand their root causes

9. B. Regular review of regulations and payer policies

10. B. Specialized codes or modifiers to specify that the service was delivered remotely

These questions are designed to reinforce key concepts in advanced billing techniques, highlighting the importance of compliance, accurate coding, and effective management of billing challenges in healthcare.

Chapter 9: Electronic Health Records (EHR) and Coding

9.1. Basics of EHR and Their Role in Coding

Electronic Health Records (EHR) have revolutionized how healthcare information is recorded, stored, and used across the healthcare industry. By transitioning from paper-based records to digital formats, EHR systems offer a comprehensive view of a patient's health history, treatments, and outcomes. This shift not only improves patient care and coordination among healthcare providers but also plays a pivotal role in the medical coding and billing process.

Understanding EHR Systems

EHR systems are digital versions of patients' paper charts, accessible in real-time and shareable among authorized healthcare providers. They contain a range of patient information, including demographics, medical history, medication and allergies, immunization status, laboratory test results, radiology images, and treatment plans.

The Role of EHR in Medical Coding

1. Enhanced Accuracy and Efficiency:

- EHR systems facilitate the accurate and efficient capture of patient encounters, reducing the likelihood of errors compared to manual coding from paper charts.

2. Improved Documentation:

- EHRs provide a structured format for documenting clinical encounters, making it easier for coders to find and use the information needed for accurate coding.

3. Integrated Coding Tools:

- Many EHR systems include integrated coding tools and databases, such as ICD-10, CPT, and HCPCS codes, enabling coders to search and enter codes directly within the patient's record.

4. Real-Time Access to Patient Data:

- Coders can access up-to-date patient information, including recent visits, diagnoses, and procedures, facilitating timely and accurate coding.

5. Streamlined Billing Process:

- EHR systems can automate certain aspects of the billing process, linking coded information directly to billing software to generate claims, which reduces manual entry and speeds up the reimbursement process.

Challenges and Considerations

1. Data Entry Errors:

- Incorrect data entry or reliance on default settings can lead to inaccuracies in patient records and coding.

2. Interoperability:

- The ability of EHR systems to communicate and exchange information seamlessly across different platforms and healthcare providers is crucial for maintaining accuracy and completeness of patient records.

3. Training and Adaptation:

- Coders and healthcare providers require training to effectively use EHR systems and coding tools, which can involve a significant investment of time and resources.

4. Privacy and Security:

- Protecting patient health information is paramount, requiring robust security measures and compliance with regulations such as HIPAA (Health Insurance Portability and Accountability Act).

Optimizing the Use of EHR in Coding

- **Continuous Training:** Regular training sessions on EHR functionalities and coding updates can enhance coding accuracy.

- **Quality Assurance:** Implementing quality checks and audits within the EHR system can help identify and correct coding errors.

- **Feedback Loops:** Creating channels for coders and clinicians to communicate effectively can improve the quality of documentation and coding.

- **Leveraging EHR Analytics:** Utilizing the data analytics capabilities of EHR systems can help identify trends in coding and documentation practices, informing areas for improvement.

Conclusion

EHR systems have become an indispensable tool in modern healthcare, significantly impacting medical coding and billing processes. By providing accurate, efficient, and accessible patient information, EHRs support the goals of improved patient care and streamlined administrative processes. Overcoming the challenges associated with EHR implementation and use requires ongoing education, collaboration, and a commitment to leveraging technology to enhance healthcare delivery and management.

9.2. Interfacing with EHR Systems

Interfacing with Electronic Health Records (EHR) systems is a critical aspect of modern healthcare, enabling seamless communication and data exchange between different healthcare software applications. This interoperability plays a pivotal role in enhancing patient care, improving efficiency, and facilitating accurate medical coding and billing.

Understanding EHR Interfacing

EHR Interfacing refers to the process of connecting disparate healthcare information systems to allow for the secure and efficient exchange of data. An interface can connect EHRs to laboratory systems, pharmacy systems, billing software, and other EHR systems across healthcare providers. This connectivity ensures that patient information is accessible and up-to-date, regardless of where treatment is being provided.

Types of EHR Interfaces

1. **Laboratory Information Systems (LIS):** Interfaces between EHRs and LIS enable the direct transfer of lab orders and results, reducing manual entry errors and improving turnaround times.

2. **Radiology Systems:** These interfaces facilitate the ordering of imaging tests directly from the EHR and the receipt of radiology

reports and images, integrating them into the patient's electronic record.

3. **Pharmacy Systems:** EHR-pharmacy interfaces allow for electronic prescribing (e-prescribing), enhancing medication accuracy and safety by reducing prescription errors.

4. **Billing Systems:** Interfaces between EHRs and medical billing software streamline the coding and billing process by automatically transferring coded data to billing systems, improving accuracy and efficiency in the revenue cycle.

5. **Health Information Exchange (HIE):** These interfaces support the sharing of patient information across different healthcare organizations and providers, improving care coordination and patient outcomes.

Benefits of EHR Interfacing

- **Improved Patient Safety:** Reduces medication and diagnostic errors by ensuring accurate and timely information transfer.

- **Enhanced Care Coordination:** Facilitates the sharing of patient data among healthcare providers, leading to better-informed treatment decisions.

- **Increased Efficiency:** Minimizes manual data entry, reducing administrative workload and the potential for errors.

- **Streamlined Billing:** Automates the transfer of coded data to billing systems, speeding up the reimbursement process.

Challenges in EHR Interfacing

- **Technical Complexity:** Developing and maintaining interfaces can be technically challenging, requiring specialized knowledge and resources.

- **Interoperability Issues:** Different EHR systems may use varying standards and formats, complicating the integration process.

- **Cost:** The development, implementation, and maintenance of interfaces can be costly, particularly for smaller healthcare providers.

- **Data Privacy and Security:** Ensuring the secure exchange of patient information across interfaces is critical, necessitating robust security measures.

Strategies for Effective EHR Interfacing

- **Adopting Standards:** Utilizing industry standards (e.g., HL7, FHIR) for data exchange can enhance interoperability between systems.

- **Collaboration:** Working with EHR vendors, interface developers, and other healthcare providers can facilitate the development of effective interfaces.

- **Comprehensive Testing:** Rigorous testing of interfaces before full implementation ensures that data exchange is accurate and secure.

- **Ongoing Training and Support:** Providing staff with training on interface functionalities and offering continuous technical support are crucial for successful interfacing.

Conclusion

Interfacing with EHR systems is essential for achieving seamless data exchange in healthcare, supporting clinical decision-making, enhancing patient care, and streamlining administrative processes. Despite the challenges, effective EHR interfacing can lead to significant improvements in healthcare delivery and patient outcomes. Ensuring successful interfacing requires a commitment to technical excellence, collaboration, and a focus on data privacy and security.

9.3. EHR and Coding Accuracy

Electronic Health Records (EHR) have a profound impact on coding accuracy, offering significant advantages over traditional paper records. By digitizing patient information, EHR systems facilitate more efficient, accurate, and streamlined coding processes, which are crucial for billing and reimbursement in healthcare settings. However, to fully leverage EHR systems for improved coding accuracy, healthcare providers must be aware of both the opportunities and challenges these systems present.

Enhancing Coding Accuracy with EHR

1. Improved Documentation:

- EHRs provide a comprehensive and detailed record of patient encounters, treatments, and outcomes, offering coders a rich source of information for accurate code assignment.

2. Integrated Coding Tools:

- Many EHR systems include built-in coding tools and databases, such as ICD-10, CPT, and HCPCS codes. These tools can suggest codes based on clinical documentation, reducing the likelihood of errors and omissions.

3. Real-Time Access and Updates:

- Coders have real-time access to patient data, allowing for timely coding of services. Furthermore, EHR systems are regularly updated to reflect the latest coding standards and guidelines, ensuring coders use the most current codes.

4. Automated Alerts and Checks:

- EHR systems can be configured to alert coders to potential errors, such as missing information or inconsistencies in documentation, which could impact code selection.

Challenges to Coding Accuracy in EHR

1. Template-Based Documentation:

- The use of templates and auto-populated fields in EHRs can lead to generic or incomplete documentation, which may not fully capture the specifics of the patient encounter, potentially affecting coding accuracy.

2. Copy and Paste Errors:

- The ease of copying and pasting within EHRs can result in duplicated or outdated information being carried over into patient records, leading to inaccuracies in coding.

3. User Training and Familiarity:

- Effective use of EHR systems for coding requires comprehensive training and familiarity with the system. Lack of proper training can hinder the ability to navigate the system efficiently and leverage its coding tools.

4. Overreliance on Automated Coding Suggestions:

- While automated coding suggestions can aid the coding process, overreliance on these features without proper review and validation can lead to coding errors.

Strategies to Maximize Coding Accuracy with EHR

1. Regular Training and Education:

- Provide ongoing training for coders and healthcare providers on the effective use of EHR systems, emphasizing the importance of accurate and thorough documentation.

2. Customization and Optimization of EHR Templates:

- Customize EHR templates to suit the specific needs of different specialties and ensure they prompt for detailed and specific documentation.

3. Rigorous Documentation Review Processes:

- Implement processes for regular review and validation of documentation within the EHR to identify and correct inaccuracies or inconsistencies.

4. Collaboration Between Clinicians and Coders:

- Encourage open communication and collaboration between clinicians and coders to clarify documentation and resolve ambiguities that could affect coding accuracy.

Conclusion

EHR systems offer significant opportunities to improve coding accuracy, which is vital for effective billing and reimbursement.

By addressing the challenges associated with EHR documentation and coding, and implementing strategies to enhance accuracy, healthcare providers can ensure that coding processes are efficient, accurate, and compliant with current standards and regulations.

9.4. Impact of EHR on Coding and Billing

The adoption of Electronic Health Records (EHR) systems has significantly impacted the landscape of medical coding and billing. EHRs have transformed how health information is captured, stored, and utilized, leading to improvements in data accuracy, efficiency in healthcare delivery, and streamlined billing processes. However, the integration of EHR systems also presents unique challenges that healthcare providers must navigate to optimize the benefits for coding and billing operations.

Positive Impacts of EHR on Coding and Billing

1. Enhanced Data Accuracy and Integrity:

- EHR systems minimize the errors associated with manual data entry and paper records. Accurate patient data is crucial for precise coding and billing, reducing the likelihood of claim denials due to incorrect information.

2. Improved Documentation for Coding:

- Comprehensive and detailed documentation in EHRs provides coders with the information needed to assign accurate codes. This includes diagnoses, procedures performed, and detailed notes on patient encounters.

3. Streamlined Billing Process:

- EHR systems can automate many aspects of the billing process, including the generation of claims based on coded data. This automation reduces the turnaround time for claim submission and can improve cash flow for healthcare providers.

4. Real-time Access to Patient Information:

- Coders and billing specialists have real-time access to patient records, enabling timely coding and billing for services rendered. This access also facilitates quick responses to queries from payers regarding claims.

5. Audit Trails for Compliance:

- EHRs provide detailed audit trails of all interactions with patient records, which is valuable for compliance purposes and in case of audits by payers. This transparency can help in defending billing decisions if questioned.

Challenges Posed by EHR Systems

1. Learning Curve and Training Requirements:

- Effective utilization of EHR systems for coding and billing requires comprehensive training for staff. The complexity and variability of EHR interfaces can present a learning curve.

2. Template and Auto-fill Drawbacks:

- While templates and auto-fill options in EHRs improve efficiency, they can also lead to generic documentation that lacks specificity, potentially affecting coding accuracy.

3. Overreliance on EHR Coding Suggestions:

- Some EHR systems offer coding suggestions based on documented information. Overreliance on these automated suggestions without proper review can result in coding errors.

4. Interoperability Issues:

- The ability of EHR systems to communicate and exchange information seamlessly with other systems (such as billing software) can vary, potentially complicating the billing process.

Strategies to Leverage EHR for Improved Coding and Billing

1. Continuous Staff Training:

- Invest in ongoing training and support for staff to ensure they are proficient in using EHR systems for coding and billing purposes.

2. Customize EHR Settings:

- Work with EHR vendors to customize templates and settings to fit the specific needs of your practice, ensuring documentation prompts are specific and relevant.

3. Implement Quality Control Measures:

- Establish quality control processes to review and validate coding and billing entries within the EHR, catching errors before claim submission.

4. Encourage Clinician-Coder Collaboration:

- Facilitate collaboration between clinicians and coders to ensure documentation is comprehensive and accurately reflects the care provided, supporting accurate coding and billing.

Conclusion

The impact of EHR systems on coding and billing is profound, offering opportunities to enhance efficiency, accuracy, and compliance. By addressing the challenges associated with EHR implementation and usage, healthcare providers can maximize the benefits of these systems, improving the overall billing process and ensuring timely reimbursement for services rendered.

9.5. Exercise: 10 MCQs with Answers at the End

Test your knowledge on the impact of Electronic Health Records (EHR) on coding and billing, including basics, interfacing, accuracy, and overall impact. Answers are provided at the end for self-assessment.

Questions

1. What is one primary benefit of EHR systems in medical coding and billing?

   A. Increased paperwork

   B. Enhanced data accuracy

   C. Reduced need for documentation

   D. Higher rates of claim denial

2. EHR systems improve documentation for coding by providing:

   A. Limited patient information

   B. Generic templates only

   C. Comprehensive and detailed records

   D. Automated coding with no need for review

3. One challenge of using EHR for coding and billing is:

   A. The impossibility of integrating with other systems

   B. The automatic reduction of coding errors to zero

   C. The learning curve and training requirements

   D. Immediate mastery by all staff members

4. In EHR systems, audit trails are important for:

   A. Only tracking patient appointments

   B. Compliance and defending billing decisions

   C. Decreasing transparency in healthcare processes

   D. Eliminating the need for coding

5. How can EHR templates potentially affect coding accuracy negatively?

   A. By providing too much detail

   B. Through generic documentation that lacks specificity

   C. By making documentation more difficult to complete

D. Templates have no impact on coding accuracy

6. Interoperability in EHR systems refers to their ability to:

  A. Operate independently without connecting to other systems

  B. Communicate and exchange information seamlessly with other healthcare software

  C. Prevent all forms of data exchange for security reasons

  D. Focus solely on billing without supporting clinical functions

7. A key strategy to leverage EHR for improved coding and billing is:

  A. Avoiding any form of staff training

  B. Disabling all automated coding suggestions

  C. Continuous staff training and support

  D. Relying solely on EHR defaults without customization

8. Overreliance on EHR coding suggestions can lead to:

  A. Perfect coding accuracy

  B. Increased efficiency with no drawbacks

  C. Coding errors without proper review

  D. Elimination of the need for coders

9. What role does clinician-coder collaboration play in EHR documentation?

   A. It is discouraged in most healthcare settings

   B. Ensures documentation is comprehensive and supports accurate coding

   C. Increases the likelihood of documentation errors

   D. Has no impact on the coding and billing process

10. Effective utilization of EHR systems for coding and billing requires:

   A. Ignoring updates to coding standards and guidelines

   B. Comprehensive training and familiarity with the system

   C. Minimal documentation of patient encounters

   D. Sole reliance on automated features without manual oversight

Answers

1. B. Enhanced data accuracy

2. C. Comprehensive and detailed records

3. C. The learning curve and training requirements

4. B. Compliance and defending billing decisions

5. B. Through generic documentation that lacks specificity

6. B. Communicate and exchange information seamlessly with other healthcare software

7. C. Continuous staff training and support

8. C. Coding errors without proper review

9. B. Ensures documentation is comprehensive and supports accurate coding

10. B. Comprehensive training and familiarity with the system

These questions underscore the importance of Electronic Health Records in modern healthcare, particularly their impact on improving coding and billing processes while highlighting potential challenges and strategies for effective utilization.

Chapter 10: Healthcare Regulations and Compliance

10.1. Understanding HIPAA and Patient Privacy

The Health Insurance Portability and Accountability Act (HIPAA) of 1996 is a pivotal piece of legislation in the United States that provides data privacy and security provisions for safeguarding medical information. Understanding HIPAA is crucial for all healthcare providers, administrators, and anyone involved in handling patient information, as it directly impacts patient privacy, healthcare operations, and the use of Electronic Health Records (EHR).

Key Provisions of HIPAA

HIPAA consists of several key provisions or "Titles" that address health insurance coverage, tax-related provisions, and, most pertinently for privacy and security, the Administrative Simplification rules. These rules are designed to protect health information while allowing the flow of data needed to provide high-quality healthcare and protect public health.

1. Privacy Rule:

- Establishes national standards for the protection of individually identifiable health information or Protected Health Information (PHI).

- Gives patients rights over their health information, including rights to examine and obtain a copy of their health records and request corrections.

2. Security Rule:

- Specifies a series of administrative, physical, and technical safeguards for covered entities to use to ensure the confidentiality, integrity, and security of electronic PHI (e-PHI).

- Requires appropriate safeguards to protect the privacy of personal health information and sets limits and conditions on the uses and disclosures that may be made of such information without patient authorization.

3. Breach Notification Rule:

- Requires covered entities and their business associates to provide notification following a breach of unsecured PHI.

Implications for Healthcare Providers

Compliance:

- Healthcare providers must ensure that all aspects of patient care and administration comply with HIPAA requirements, including the secure handling, storage, and transmission of PHI.

Training and Policies:

- Providers must implement privacy policies, conduct regular training for employees, and ensure that everyone in the organization understands their role in protecting patient privacy.

Patient Rights:

- Facilities must inform patients about their privacy rights under HIPAA, including how their information can be used and shared.

Challenges and Considerations

1. Technology and Security:

- The increasing use of digital health records and telehealth services presents ongoing challenges in securing e-PHI, requiring up-to-date security measures and continuous vigilance.

2. Third-Party Business Associates:

- HIPAA compliance extends to all business associates that handle PHI on behalf of a healthcare provider. Ensuring that third parties adhere to HIPAA standards is essential for comprehensive compliance.

3. State Laws:

- In some cases, state laws may provide more stringent privacy protections than HIPAA. Healthcare providers must navigate both federal and state regulations to ensure full legal compliance.

Strategies for Ensuring HIPAA Compliance

- **Conduct Regular Risk Assessments:** Identify potential vulnerabilities in the handling and storage of PHI and implement measures to mitigate these risks.

- **Implement Strong Data Encryption:** Use encryption for storing and transmitting e-PHI to protect against unauthorized access.

- **Develop Clear Policies and Procedures:** Create detailed policies for managing PHI, including procedures for responding to data breaches.

- **Train Staff Regularly:** Provide ongoing training to all employees on HIPAA regulations and the importance of patient privacy.

Conclusion

HIPAA plays a fundamental role in shaping the practices of healthcare providers regarding patient privacy and the handling of health information. Adhering to HIPAA not only ensures compliance but also builds trust with patients by safeguarding their personal health information. As healthcare continues to evolve, particularly with advances in technology, maintaining HIPAA compliance remains a dynamic and critical priority for the healthcare industry.

10.2. Fraud, Abuse, and Compliance in Coding

Fraud and abuse in medical coding and billing are significant concerns within the healthcare industry, leading to billions of dollars in losses annually for federal healthcare programs like Medicare and Medicaid, as well as for private insurers. These practices not only result in financial losses but also undermine the integrity of the healthcare system and can negatively impact patient care. Understanding the distinction between fraud and abuse, recognizing their indicators, and adhering to compliance standards are crucial for preventing these illicit activities.

Defining Fraud and Abuse

Fraud involves intentional deception or misrepresentation that an individual knows to be false, or does not believe to be true, and makes, knowing that the deception could result in some unauthorized benefit to himself/herself or some other person. Examples include billing for services not rendered, falsifying a patient's diagnosis to justify unnecessary tests, and knowingly billing for services at a higher level than provided or necessary.

Abuse refers to practices that are inconsistent with sound fiscal, business, or medical practices, and result in unnecessary costs to healthcare programs, or in reimbursement for services that are not medically necessary or that fail to meet professionally recognized standards for healthcare. It also includes practices that are not necessarily fraudulent but are improper.

Indicators of Fraud and Abuse

- Billing for services not rendered.

- Upcoding services or procedures (billing for a more expensive service than the one actually provided).

- Unbundling (billing each step of a procedure as if it were a separate procedure).

- Providing medically unnecessary services.

- Misrepresenting non-covered treatments as medically necessary covered treatments for the purpose of obtaining insurance payments.

- Kickbacks and bribery for patient referrals.

Compliance in Coding

Compliance programs are essential for preventing fraud and abuse in medical coding and billing. These programs typically include:

- **Regular Training and Education:** Ensuring that coding and billing staff are well-informed about the latest coding standards, regulatory requirements, and ethical practices.

- **Internal Audits and Monitoring:** Conducting regular audits of coding practices and billing records to identify and rectify any inaccuracies or inconsistencies.

- **Clear Policies and Procedures:** Developing and enforcing clear policies regarding coding and billing practices, including disciplinary measures for violations.

- **Open Lines of Communication:** Establishing channels through which staff can report suspected fraud or abuse without fear of retaliation.

Legal and Regulatory Framework

Several laws and regulations address fraud and abuse in healthcare, including:

- **The False Claims Act (FCA):** Prohibits submitting false or fraudulent claims for payment to the federal government.

- **The Anti-Kickback Statute:** Prohibits offering, paying, soliciting, or receiving remuneration to induce referrals of items or services covered by federally funded programs.

- **The Stark Law:** Prohibits physicians from referring patients to receive "designated health services" payable by Medicare or Medicaid from entities with which the physician or an immediate family member has a financial relationship, unless an exception applies.

Conclusion

Fraud and abuse in medical coding and billing not only pose legal risks but also erode trust in the healthcare system. Implementing robust compliance programs, staying informed about legal standards, and fostering an organizational culture of integrity and accountability are vital steps in combating these practices. Through diligent efforts, healthcare providers can help ensure that coding and billing practices are accurate, ethical, and in full compliance with applicable laws and regulations.

10.3. Navigating Healthcare Laws and Regulations

Healthcare laws and regulations in the United States are complex and multifaceted, designed to ensure patient safety, protect public health, and promote ethical practices within the healthcare industry. For healthcare providers and organizations, navigating these laws and regulations is essential for compliance, avoiding legal liabilities, and maintaining the trust of patients and the public. This comprehensive overview explores key areas of healthcare regulation and offers strategies for effective navigation and compliance.

Key Areas of Healthcare Regulation

1. Patient Privacy and Data Security:

- HIPAA (Health Insurance Portability and Accountability Act): Protects patient health information, ensuring data privacy and security.

- **HITECH Act (Health Information Technology for Economic and Clinical Health):** Expands HIPAA rules, especially in the context of electronic health records (EHRs), and increases penalties for non-compliance.

2. Fraud, Waste, and Abuse Prevention:

- **False Claims Act:** Prohibits knowingly submitting false claims to federal healthcare programs.

- **Anti-Kickback Statute:** Makes it illegal to offer, pay, solicit, or receive remuneration to induce referrals of items or services covered by federal healthcare programs.

- **Stark Law:** Addresses physician self-referral, prohibiting physicians from referring patients to entities with which they have a financial relationship.

3. Quality of Care and Patient Safety:

- **Affordable Care Act (ACA):** Includes provisions to improve the quality of care, expand access to insurance, and increase consumer protections.

- **Patient Safety and Quality Improvement Act:** Establishes a voluntary reporting system for patient safety events to enhance data collection and analysis for improving patient safety outcomes.

4. Licensure and Credentialing:

- State-specific laws regulate the licensure of healthcare professionals and the accreditation of healthcare facilities, ensuring that providers meet certain standards of practice.

Strategies for Navigating Healthcare Laws and Regulations

1. Establish a Compliance Program:

- Develop and implement a comprehensive compliance program that addresses key regulatory areas, including patient privacy, fraud prevention, and quality of care.

2. Continuous Education and Training:

- Regularly educate and train staff on relevant laws and regulations, compliance policies, and ethical practices to ensure everyone is informed and compliant.

3. Stay Informed:

- Keep up-to-date with changes in healthcare laws and regulations through subscriptions to regulatory updates, membership in professional organizations, and attendance at industry conferences.

4. Conduct Regular Audits:

- Perform routine audits and risk assessments to identify potential areas of non-compliance or vulnerability and take corrective action as necessary.

5. Foster a Culture of Compliance and Ethics:

- Promote an organizational culture that values adherence to legal standards, ethical practices, and transparency, encouraging staff to report concerns without fear of retaliation.

6. Seek Expert Advice:

- Consult with legal and regulatory experts, especially when navigating complex compliance issues or responding to regulatory inquiries and investigations.

Conclusion

Navigating the complex landscape of healthcare laws and regulations is a critical responsibility for healthcare providers and organizations. By implementing robust compliance strategies, staying informed about legal requirements, and fostering a culture of ethics and transparency, healthcare entities can mitigate risks, enhance patient care, and uphold the integrity of the healthcare system.

10.4. The Role of Compliance in Medical Coding

Compliance in medical coding is a critical aspect of healthcare administration, ensuring that coding practices adhere to legal and regulatory standards. It serves as a safeguard against fraudulent billing practices, mitigates the risk of audits and penalties, and ensures accurate reimbursement for healthcare services. The role of compliance in medical coding cannot be overstated, as it directly impacts the financial health of healthcare organizations and maintains the integrity of the healthcare system.

Importance of Compliance in Medical Coding

1. Ensures Accurate Reimbursement:

- Proper coding is essential for healthcare providers to receive appropriate payment for services rendered. Compliance ensures that codes accurately reflect the care provided, based on documentation.

2. Prevents Fraud and Abuse:

- Compliance programs help prevent intentional billing for services not provided, upcoding, and other fraudulent activities that can lead to legal action and financial penalties.

3. Reduces the Risk of Audits and Penalties:

- Adhering to coding standards minimizes the risk of audits by Medicare, Medicaid, and other payers. Compliance reduces the likelihood of findings of improper billing, thereby avoiding fines and penalties.

4. Maintains Integrity and Trust:

- Compliance in coding practices demonstrates a commitment to ethical behavior, building trust among patients, payers, and regulatory bodies.

Key Components of a Coding Compliance Program

1. Policies and Procedures:

- Develop clear, written policies and procedures that outline coding practices, compliance standards, and the handling of discrepancies or errors.

2. Education and Training:

- Provide ongoing education and training for coding staff, clinicians, and billing personnel on current coding guidelines, payer policies, and regulatory updates.

3. Regular Audits and Monitoring:

- Conduct regular internal audits to review coding accuracy and compliance with policies. Use audit findings to identify areas for improvement and implement corrective actions.

4. Enforcement and Disciplinary Guidelines:

- Establish enforcement mechanisms and disciplinary guidelines for non-compliance with coding standards. Ensure that staff understand the consequences of non-compliance.

5. Open Lines of Communication:

- Create channels for staff to report concerns or questions related to coding practices without fear of retaliation. Encourage a culture of transparency and openness.

Challenges in Ensuring Coding Compliance

1. Evolving Regulations and Guidelines:

- Keeping up with constant changes in coding guidelines, payer policies, and regulations can be challenging for healthcare organizations.

2. Complexity of Medical Services:

- The complexity of medical procedures and the nuances of coding rules can make accurate coding challenging, increasing the risk of errors.

3. Resource Limitations:

- Small healthcare providers may lack the resources to implement comprehensive compliance programs or conduct regular training and audits.

Strategies for Enhancing Coding Compliance

1. Leverage Technology:

- Utilize advanced coding software and EHR systems with built-in compliance checks and alerts to assist coders and reduce errors.

2. Foster a Culture of Compliance:

- Promote a culture where compliance is viewed as everyone's responsibility. Recognize and reward compliance and ethical behavior.

3. Seek External Expertise:

- Consider consulting with external experts or outsourcing certain compliance functions to specialists, particularly for complex coding issues or audit preparations.

Conclusion

Compliance in medical coding is foundational to the ethical and financial integrity of healthcare organizations. By implementing robust compliance programs, healthcare providers can ensure accurate coding, prevent fraudulent practices, and maintain trust with patients and payers. Embracing continuous education, leveraging technology, and fostering a culture of compliance are key to navigating the complexities of medical coding in today's healthcare environment.

10.5. Exercise: 10 MCQs with Answers at the End

Test your knowledge on healthcare regulations and compliance, including HIPAA, fraud and abuse prevention, navigating healthcare laws, and the role of compliance in medical coding. Answers are provided at the end for self-assessment.

Questions

1. What does HIPAA primarily protect?

   A. Healthcare provider incomes

   B. Patient health information

   C. Insurance company profits

   D. Hospital parking regulations

2. The False Claims Act is aimed at:

   A. Reducing paperwork in healthcare

   B. Preventing fraudulent billing to federal healthcare programs

   C. Encouraging the use of generic drugs

   D. Lowering healthcare costs through technology

3. Which of the following is considered healthcare fraud?

A. Billing for services not rendered

B. Using ICD-10 codes accurately

C. Implementing an EHR system

D. Providing free healthcare services

4. The Anti-Kickback Statute prohibits:

A. Referrals to specialists

B. Kickbacks for patient referrals

C. Accepting gifts from patients

D. Billing for preventive care services

5. A compliance program in medical coding should NOT include:

A. Regular audits and monitoring

B. Policies that encourage upcoding

C. Education and training on coding standards

D. Open lines of communication for reporting concerns

6. The primary purpose of coding audits is to:

A. Punish coders for mistakes

B. Ensure accuracy and compliance in coding practices

C. Reduce the workload of medical coders

D. Increase the revenue of healthcare providers

7. HIPAA's Privacy Rule gives patients the right to:

    A. Choose any healthcare provider without restrictions

    B. Obtain a copy of their medical records

    C. Bill their insurance directly

    D. Receive all healthcare services for free

8. The HITECH Act expands rules on:

    A. Hospital construction standards

    B. Electronic health records and patient data security

    C. The use of medical devices

    D. Healthcare provider licensing

9. Compliance with healthcare regulations is important for:

    A. Only large healthcare institutions

    B. Every healthcare provider and organization

    C. Solely outpatient clinics

    D. Only those dealing with Medicare and Medicaid

10. Stark Law addresses:

   A. The minimum number of hospital beds required

   B. Physician self-referral for certain designated health services

   C. The color coding of medical records

   D. Restrictions on pharmaceutical advertising

Answers

1. B. Patient health information

2. B. Preventing fraudulent billing to federal healthcare programs

3. A. Billing for services not rendered

4. B. Kickbacks for patient referrals

5. B. Policies that encourage upcoding

6. B. Ensure accuracy and compliance in coding practices

7. B. Obtain a copy of their medical records

8. B. Electronic health records and patient data security

9. B. Every healthcare provider and organization

10. B. Physician self-referral for certain designated health services

These questions and answers are designed to reinforce your understanding of critical aspects of healthcare regulations and compliance, highlighting the importance of protecting patient information, preventing fraud, and ensuring accurate coding practices within the healthcare industry.

Chapter 11: Specialty Coding I: Outpatient Services

11.1. Coding for Outpatient Services

Outpatient services encompass a wide range of medical treatments and procedures that do not require an overnight hospital stay. These services can include routine check-ups, minor surgeries, diagnostic tests, emergency department visits, and therapy sessions, among others. Coding for outpatient services involves specific considerations and guidelines to accurately capture the scope and nature of the care provided.

Key Aspects of Outpatient Coding

1. CPT Codes:

- The Current Procedural Terminology (CPT) codes are primarily used for coding outpatient services. These codes describe medical, surgical, and diagnostic services and are crucial for billing purposes and statistical analysis.

2. HCPCS Level II Codes:

- For services, procedures, and supplies not covered by CPT codes, Healthcare Common Procedure Coding System (HCPCS)

Level II codes are used. This includes durable medical equipment (DME), prosthetics, ambulance rides, and certain drugs and medicines.

3. ICD-10-CM Codes:

- The International Classification of Diseases, Tenth Revision, Clinical Modification (ICD-10-CM) codes are used to document the patient's diagnosis and are essential for supporting the medical necessity of the services provided.

Coding Guidelines for Outpatient Services

Accurate and Specific Documentation:

- Documentation must clearly detail the services provided, including the extent and complexity of care, to support the selected codes.

Use of Modifiers:

- Modifiers are used with CPT and HCPCS codes to indicate specific circumstances of the services provided, such as bilateral procedures, multiple procedures, or services that are part of a global surgery package.

Understanding Payer Policies:

- It's crucial to be aware of the specific coding and billing guidelines of various insurance payers, as policies can differ significantly.

Awareness of Global Surgery Rules:

- Certain procedures have global periods during which postoperative care is included in the payment for the initial procedure. Understanding these rules is essential for accurate coding of follow-up care.

Challenges in Outpatient Coding

Keeping Up with Changes:

- CPT, HCPCS, and ICD-10-CM codes are updated annually, requiring coders to stay current with the latest revisions and guidelines.

Complexity of Services:

- The wide range of services and treatments in the outpatient setting can make coding complex, especially when multiple procedures are performed during a single visit.

Payer-Specific Requirements:

- Navigating the diverse and sometimes conflicting requirements of different insurance payers adds complexity to the coding process.

Strategies for Effective Outpatient Coding

Continuous Education and Training:

- Regular training sessions and professional development opportunities can help coders stay informed about coding updates and best practices.

Utilization of Coding Software:

- Advanced coding software can assist in selecting the appropriate codes and identifying potential errors before claim submission.

Quality Assurance Processes:

- Implementing quality checks and audits of coded data can help ensure accuracy and compliance with coding standards and payer policies.

Collaboration with Healthcare Providers:

- Effective communication and collaboration between coders and healthcare providers are essential for clarifying documentation and ensuring that all services are accurately coded.

Conclusion

Coding for outpatient services is a dynamic and integral part of the healthcare revenue cycle. By adhering to coding guidelines, staying informed about updates, and implementing effective strategies to address challenges, coders can ensure accurate representation of outpatient services. This not only supports the financial health of healthcare organizations but also contributes to the overall quality of patient care.

11.2. Challenges in Outpatient Coding

Outpatient coding is a crucial aspect of medical coding, requiring precision and a deep understanding of various coding systems and payer policies. However, professionals in this field often encounter several challenges that can complicate the coding process, impact reimbursement, and increase the risk of audits. Identifying and addressing these challenges is essential for maintaining accuracy, compliance, and efficiency in outpatient coding.

Common Challenges in Outpatient Coding

1. Frequent Changes in Coding Guidelines:

- The coding guidelines for CPT, HCPCS, and ICD-10-CM codes undergo regular updates and revisions. Keeping up with these changes can be daunting and requires continuous education and adaptation.

2. Documentation Issues:

- Inadequate or unclear documentation from healthcare providers can significantly hinder the coding process. Coders often face challenges in determining the appropriate codes due to missing information or nonspecific documentation.

3. Complex Payer Policies:

- Insurance companies have their own specific billing requirements and coverage policies. Navigating these diverse and sometimes conflicting policies can be challenging and time-consuming for coders.

4. Use of Modifiers:

- Correctly applying modifiers is essential for accurate outpatient coding. However, understanding and remembering the specific circumstances under which to use each modifier can be difficult, leading to errors and potential claim denials.

5. High Volume of Services:

- Outpatient settings typically see a high volume of patients and a wide variety of services, which can be overwhelming for coders, especially in facilities with limited staffing resources.

6. Technology and Software Limitations:

- While electronic health records (EHR) and coding software can facilitate the coding process, technical issues, software limitations, or a lack of integration can pose significant challenges.

7. Compliance and Audit Risks:

- Ensuring compliance with all regulatory requirements and minimizing the risk of audits is a constant concern. Incorrect coding or failure to adhere to guidelines can result in financial penalties and legal issues.

Strategies for Overcoming Challenges

1. Ongoing Education and Training:

- Regular training sessions, webinars, and workshops can help coders stay current with coding changes and payer policies.

2. Effective Communication with Healthcare Providers:

- Establishing clear channels of communication between coders and providers can improve the quality of documentation and clarify ambiguities.

3. Utilization of Coding Resources and Tools:

- Leveraging coding manuals, online resources, and software tools can aid in accurate code selection and modifier application.

4. Quality Assurance Measures:

- Implementing regular audits and quality checks can identify coding inaccuracies and areas for improvement, reducing the risk of compliance issues.

5. Collaboration and Teamwork:

- Encouraging teamwork and collaboration among coding staff can help distribute the workload, share knowledge, and solve complex coding issues.

6. Advocating for Technology Improvements:

- Working with IT departments or software vendors to address technology limitations and enhance EHR and coding software functionalities can improve coding efficiency.

Conclusion

Outpatient coding presents a set of unique challenges that require a proactive and informed approach to manage effectively. By investing in education, leveraging technology, and fostering communication and collaboration, coding professionals can overcome these challenges, ensuring accurate, compliant, and efficient coding practices in outpatient settings.

11.3. Outpatient Surgery Coding

Outpatient surgery coding involves the accurate representation of surgical procedures performed without the need for an overnight hospital stay. These surgeries can range from minor procedures to more complex operations, all conducted in ambulatory surgery centers (ASCs), outpatient departments of hospitals, or specialized clinics. The precision of coding in this setting is critical, not only for appropriate reimbursement but also for ensuring patient records accurately reflect the care provided.

Key Considerations for Outpatient Surgery Coding

1. CPT Codes:

- The Current Procedural Terminology (CPT) is the primary coding system used for documenting outpatient surgeries. It provides a uniform language for describing surgical, medical, and diagnostic services.

2. Use of Modifiers:

- Modifiers play a crucial role in outpatient surgery coding, offering additional details about the procedure performed. They can indicate whether a procedure was bilateral, involved multiple procedures, was repeated, or was part of a global surgical package.

3. Documentation Requirements:

- Accurate coding relies heavily on detailed surgical reports and physician documentation. Coders must ensure that documentation clearly describes the procedure, including the surgical approach, any complications, and the outcome.

4. Facility vs. Professional Coding:

- In outpatient settings, there's often a distinction between facility coding (for the use of the facility, equipment, and supplies) and professional coding (for the services provided by the surgeon and anesthesiologist). Understanding how to navigate both is essential for accurate billing.

Challenges in Outpatient Surgery Coding

1. Complex Procedures:

- Some outpatient surgeries involve complex, multi-step procedures that can be challenging to code accurately, especially when multiple CPT codes may apply.

2. Staying Current with Coding Updates:

- The CPT code set is updated annually, requiring coders to stay informed about new, revised, and deleted codes relevant to outpatient surgery.

3. Distinguishing Between Inpatient and Outpatient Procedures:

- Certain procedures can be performed in both inpatient and outpatient settings. Coders must carefully consider the setting to choose the correct codes.

4. Identifying Bundled Services:

- The concept of bundled services, where certain pre-, intra-, and post-operative services are included in a single procedure code, can be a source of confusion and coding errors.

Strategies for Effective Outpatient Surgery Coding

1. Continuous Education and Training:

- Coders should engage in ongoing education to keep up with changes in CPT codes and guidelines, focusing on those specific to outpatient surgery.

2. Thorough Review of Documentation:

- Careful review of surgical reports and physician notes is critical. Coders should seek clarification from the surgeon if the documentation is unclear or incomplete.

3. Utilize Coding Resources:

- Access to comprehensive coding manuals, online resources, and professional coding advisories can help coders resolve complex coding issues.

4. Collaborate with Healthcare Providers:

- Establishing a collaborative relationship with surgeons and other healthcare providers supports accurate documentation and coding. Providers can offer insights into the nuances of surgical procedures that impact coding.

5. Regular Audits:

- Conducting regular coding audits can identify patterns of errors or inconsistencies, providing opportunities for corrective action and education.

Conclusion

Outpatient surgery coding is a detailed and dynamic aspect of medical coding that requires a high level of expertise and constant vigilance to changes in coding standards. By focusing on education, thorough documentation review, and effective use of coding resources, coders can achieve accurate and compliant coding for outpatient surgeries, thereby supporting the financial health of healthcare organizations and ensuring the integrity of patient records.

11.4. Outpatient Diagnostic Coding

Outpatient diagnostic coding involves assigning codes to diagnoses, symptoms, conditions, and procedures documented during outpatient visits. This coding is crucial for patient records, billing, and insurance reimbursement. Accurate diagnostic coding in the outpatient setting supports effective patient care management, facilitates health statistics tracking, and ensures healthcare providers are reimbursed appropriately for their services.

Key Aspects of Outpatient Diagnostic Coding

1. ICD-10-CM Codes:

- The International Classification of Diseases, Tenth Revision, Clinical Modification (ICD-10-CM) is the standard coding system used for diagnoses in outpatient settings. It provides detailed codes to represent patients' symptoms, diseases, and conditions.

2. Focus on the Chief Complaint:

- Outpatient coding primarily focuses on the reason for the visit or the chief complaint, along with any additional relevant diagnoses identified during the visit.

3. Linking Diagnoses to Procedures:

- Accurate outpatient diagnostic coding requires linking each procedure performed to a corresponding diagnosis code to justify the medical necessity of the procedure.

Challenges in Outpatient Diagnostic Coding

1. Documentation Quality:

- Incomplete or nonspecific documentation can significantly challenge accurate diagnostic coding. Coders often rely on thorough documentation to select the most accurate ICD-10-CM codes.

2. Keeping Up with ICD-10-CM Updates:

- The ICD-10-CM codes are updated annually, introducing new codes, revising existing ones, and sometimes deleting outdated codes. Coders need to stay current with these changes to ensure coding accuracy.

3. High Volume of Patient Visits:

- Outpatient facilities often experience a high volume of patient visits, each requiring diagnostic coding. Managing this volume without sacrificing coding accuracy can be challenging.

4. Understanding Clinical Terminology:

- A deep understanding of clinical terminology and conditions is essential for coders to accurately interpret medical records and apply the correct ICD-10-CM codes.

Strategies for Effective Outpatient Diagnostic Coding

1. Regular Training and Education:

- Ongoing education on ICD-10-CM updates and coding best practices is crucial. Coders should also be trained in clinical terminology and pathology to improve coding accuracy.

2. Utilize Coding Resources and Software:

- Access to up-to-date coding manuals, online resources, and coding software can help coders find and verify codes quickly and efficiently.

3. Quality Documentation Practices:

- Encouraging healthcare providers to produce detailed, specific, and clear documentation supports more accurate diagnostic coding.

4. Implement Quality Assurance Processes:

- Regular audits and quality checks of coded data help identify patterns of errors or areas for improvement, facilitating continuous coding accuracy enhancement.

5. Collaboration Between Coders and Healthcare Providers:

- Fostering open communication and collaboration between coders and healthcare providers can clarify ambiguous documentation and ensure the selection of appropriate diagnostic codes.

Conclusion

Outpatient diagnostic coding is a foundational component of healthcare billing and record-keeping, requiring meticulous attention to detail and a comprehensive understanding of coding standards and medical terminology. By adopting effective strategies to address common challenges, healthcare organizations can enhance coding accuracy, streamline the billing process, and ultimately support the delivery of high-quality patient care.

11.5. Exercise: 10 MCQs with Answers at the End

Test your understanding of Specialty Coding I: Outpatient Services, including the nuances of coding for outpatient services, surgeries, diagnostics, and the related challenges and strategies. Answers are provided at the end for self-assessment.

Questions

1. What coding system is primarily used for documenting outpatient diagnostic services?

   A. ICD-10-CM

   B. CPT

   C. HCPCS Level II

   D. ICD-10-PCS

2. Which of the following best describes the focus of outpatient diagnostic coding?

   A. Only the procedures performed

   B. The patient's family medical history

   C. The reason for the visit or chief complaint

   D. All medications prescribed during the visit

3. Modifiers in outpatient coding are used to indicate:

   A. Only services provided by nurses

   B. Specific circumstances surrounding a procedure

   C. The patient's income level

   D. The healthcare provider's specialty

4. Challenges in outpatient surgery coding often include:

A. Simplified procedures that require minimal coding

B. Lack of any need for documentation

C. Complex procedures that involve multiple steps

D. Procedures that do not require coding

5. What is essential for linking diagnoses to procedures in outpatient coding?

A. Guesswork based on common practices

B. A high volume of patient visits

C. Justifying the medical necessity of the procedure

D. The use of only primary diagnosis codes

6. A significant challenge in outpatient diagnostic coding is:

A. The infrequent updates to the ICD-10-CM codes

B. Keeping up with annual ICD-10-CM updates

C. The lack of available codes for common outpatient services

D. The requirement to use only handwritten documentation

7. Effective strategies for outpatient coding include:

A. Ignoring coding updates and guidelines

B. Regular training and education on coding standards

C. Avoiding communication with healthcare providers

D. Using outdated coding manuals

8. The primary role of quality documentation practices in outpatient coding is to:

A. Reduce the workload of healthcare providers

B. Support more accurate diagnostic coding

C. Completely automate the coding process

D. Increase the number of patient visits

9. In outpatient surgery coding, facility vs. professional coding distinction is important because:

A. It helps in determining the patient's eligibility for surgery

B. It separates coding for the use of facility resources from services provided by medical professionals

C. All outpatient surgeries are coded only as professional services

D. Facility codes are used exclusively for inpatient procedures

10. Continuous education and training in outpatient coding are crucial for:

A. Maintaining a static approach to coding practices

B. Keeping coders and billing staff updated on coding changes and payer policies

C. Ensuring that all coding is done manually

D. Decreasing the overall accuracy of coding

Answers

1. A. ICD-10-CM

2. C. The reason for the visit or chief complaint

3. B. Specific circumstances surrounding a procedure

4. C. Complex procedures that involve multiple steps

5. C. Justifying the medical necessity of the procedure

6. B. Keeping up with annual ICD-10-CM updates

7. B. Regular training and education on coding standards

8. B. Support more accurate diagnostic coding

9. B. It separates coding for the use of facility resources from services provided by medical professionals

10. B. Keeping coders and billing staff updated on coding changes and payer policies

These questions and answers aim to reinforce key concepts related to outpatient services coding, emphasizing the importance of accurate documentation, continuous learning, and the challenges faced in ensuring precise and compliant coding practices.

Chapter 12: Specialty Coding II: Inpatient Services

12.1. Inpatient Coding Basics

Inpatient coding refers to the process of documenting medical services provided to patients who are admitted to a hospital or healthcare facility for treatment that requires at least one overnight stay. This coding is crucial for hospital reimbursement, patient care management, and the compilation of health statistics. Unlike outpatient coding, inpatient coding focuses on capturing the entirety of a patient's encounter, from admission to discharge, using specific coding systems.

Key Coding Systems for Inpatient Services

1. ICD-10-CM for Diagnoses:

- The International Classification of Diseases, Tenth Revision, Clinical Modification (ICD-10-CM) is used for documenting diagnoses. Inpatient coders must capture all relevant diagnoses that affect the patient's care and treatment outcomes.

2. ICD-10-PCS for Procedures:

- The International Classification of Diseases, Tenth Revision, Procedure Coding System (ICD-10-PCS) is exclusively used in the inpatient setting for documenting procedures. This system provides a high level of specificity and detail, reflecting the services provided during the hospital stay.

Principles of Inpatient Coding

Principal Diagnosis:

- The principal diagnosis is the condition that, after study, is established as chiefly responsible for the patient's admission to the hospital. Identifying the principal diagnosis is crucial for determining the DRG (Diagnosis-Related Group).

Secondary Diagnoses:

- These are additional conditions that coexist at the time of admission, develop during the stay, or affect the treatment received and the length of stay. Coding secondary diagnoses can impact DRG assignment and reimbursement.

Procedure Coding:

- All significant procedures performed during the inpatient stay are coded using ICD-10-PCS codes. Accurate procedure coding is essential for DRG assignment and appropriate reimbursement.

Challenges in Inpatient Coding

Complexity of Cases:

- Inpatient cases often involve complex medical conditions and treatments, requiring a deep understanding of medical terminology, anatomy, and coding guidelines.

DRG Assignment:

- Determining the correct DRG, which impacts reimbursement rates, can be challenging due to the complexities of coding and the specifics of each case.

Documentation Quality:

- Inadequate or unclear documentation from healthcare providers can hinder accurate coding, leading to potential issues with reimbursement and compliance.

Strategies for Effective Inpatient Coding

Continuous Education and Training:

- Ongoing training on ICD-10-CM and ICD-10-PCS updates, as well as DRG guidelines, is essential for maintaining coding accuracy.

Collaboration with Healthcare Providers:

- Coders should work closely with physicians and other healthcare providers to ensure comprehensive and accurate documentation of patient care.

Quality Assurance Programs:

- Implementing quality checks and audits helps identify coding errors or inconsistencies, allowing for corrective actions and improvements.

Use of Coding Resources:

- Coders should utilize available coding manuals, online resources, and software tools to assist with accurate code assignment and DRG determination.

Conclusion

Inpatient coding plays a vital role in the healthcare reimbursement system, directly influencing hospital revenue and patient care outcomes. By adhering to coding guidelines, staying informed about updates, and implementing effective strategies to address challenges, inpatient coders can ensure accurate and compliant documentation of hospital services.

12.2. Coding for Complex Inpatient Cases

Coding for complex inpatient cases presents a unique set of challenges, requiring a deep understanding of medical terminology, disease processes, and the intricacies of coding systems. These cases often involve patients with multiple diagnoses, extensive procedures, and prolonged hospital stays, making accurate and comprehensive coding essential for proper reimbursement and patient care documentation.

Key Considerations in Coding Complex Inpatient Cases

1. Principal and Secondary Diagnoses:

- Identifying the principal diagnosis, the condition chiefly responsible for the patient's hospital stay, is crucial. Equally important is accurately coding all relevant secondary diagnoses that impact the patient's care, length of stay, and resource utilization.

2. Procedure Coding with ICD-10-PCS:

- Complex inpatient cases may involve multiple surgical or medical procedures. Each procedure must be coded accurately using ICD-10-PCS, requiring coders to understand the specifics of each procedure, including approach, device used, and any qualifiers.

3. Comorbidities and Complications (CC) and Major Comorbidities and Complications (MCC):

- Correctly identifying CCs and MCCs is essential for DRG (Diagnosis-Related Group) assignment. These conditions can significantly affect the severity level of the DRG, impacting reimbursement.

4. Use of Clinical Documentation Improvement (CDI) Programs:

- CDI programs play a vital role in ensuring the completeness and accuracy of medical documentation, facilitating precise coding and optimal DRG assignment.

Challenges in Coding Complex Inpatient Cases

1. Detailed Documentation Requirement:

- The need for detailed and specific documentation to support coding choices can be challenging, especially when documentation is incomplete or lacks clarity.

2. Staying Updated with Coding Guidelines:

- Coding guidelines, particularly for ICD-10-PCS, are complex and frequently updated. Keeping abreast of these changes is crucial for accurate coding.

3. DRG Assignment and Reimbursement Implications:

- Determining the correct DRG for complex cases can be difficult but is critical for ensuring appropriate reimbursement. Errors in DRG assignment can lead to significant financial losses or audits.

4. Interdisciplinary Collaboration:

- Effective communication and collaboration among coders, physicians, and other healthcare professionals are essential but can be challenging to achieve consistently.

Strategies for Effective Coding of Complex Inpatient Cases

1. Continuous Education and Training:

- Ongoing education for coders on the latest coding guidelines, medical terminologies, and clinical knowledge is essential for handling complex cases.

2. Implementing or Enhancing CDI Programs:

- A robust CDI program can help improve the quality of clinical documentation, making it easier for coders to assign accurate codes and DRGs.

3. Regular Audits and Feedback Loops:

- Conducting regular coding audits and providing feedback to coders and clinicians can help identify and correct coding issues, reducing errors and improving documentation.

4. Leveraging Technology:

- Utilizing advanced coding software and EHR systems that offer coding assistance, alerts for potential errors, and access to up-to-date coding guidelines can enhance coding accuracy.

5. Promoting Interdisciplinary Collaboration:

- Encouraging regular communication and collaboration between coders, physicians, and other healthcare providers ensures that documentation accurately reflects the care provided, supporting appropriate coding.

Conclusion

Coding for complex inpatient cases requires a meticulous approach, deep clinical and coding knowledge, and effective collaboration across the healthcare team. By adopting strategic practices such as continuous education, leveraging technology, and enhancing clinical documentation, healthcare facilities can navigate the challenges of coding complex cases, ensuring accurate documentation, optimal reimbursement, and high-quality patient care.

12.3. DRG and Inpatient Reimbursement

Diagnosis-Related Groups (DRGs) are a pivotal component of the inpatient reimbursement system in many healthcare systems, including Medicare and Medicaid in the United States. DRGs categorize hospital cases into groups that are clinically similar and expected to consume similar levels of hospital resources, thereby standardizing payments to hospitals for inpatient stays. Understanding DRGs is essential for healthcare providers to ensure accurate billing and optimal reimbursement for inpatient services.

Basics of the DRG System

1. Classification:

- Patients are classified into DRGs based on their principal diagnosis, secondary diagnoses (comorbidities and complications), surgical procedures performed, age, sex, and discharge status. Each DRG has a payment weight assigned to it, based on the average resources used to treat patients in that group.

2. DRG Payment Model:

- The DRG payment model is prospective, meaning the hospital is paid a predetermined amount for each inpatient stay, regardless of the actual cost incurred. This system incentivizes hospitals to manage resources efficiently while maintaining quality care.

Key Factors Influencing DRG Assignment

- **Principal Diagnosis:** The main condition treated during the hospital stay.

- **Secondary Diagnoses:** Conditions that coexist at the time of admission or develop during the stay, which may affect patient care.

- **Procedures Performed:** Surgical or medical interventions undertaken during the hospital stay.

- **Patient Demographics:** Age and sex can influence DRG assignment due to differences in resource use.

- **Discharge Status:** Whether the patient was discharged to home, another hospital, or a long-term care facility.

Challenges with DRG Assignment

- **Documentation Quality:** Inadequate or inaccurate documentation can lead to incorrect DRG assignment, impacting reimbursement.

- **Complexity of Cases:** Patients with multiple comorbidities or those undergoing numerous procedures can complicate DRG assignment.

- **Regulatory Changes:** DRG classifications and reimbursement rates are subject to change, requiring hospitals to stay updated on the latest guidelines.

Strategies for Optimizing DRG Assignment and Reimbursement

1. Clinical Documentation Improvement (CDI):

- Implementing a robust CDI program can enhance the quality of clinical documentation, ensuring that it accurately reflects the patient's condition and the care provided.

2. Regular Training for Coders and Clinicians:

- Ongoing education on the importance of accurate documentation and coding practices can help improve DRG assignment accuracy.

3. Utilization Review:

- Conducting reviews of patient records prior to discharge can identify any discrepancies or missing information that could affect DRG assignment.

4. Technology and Software Solutions:

- Leveraging advanced coding and documentation software can assist in identifying potential DRG optimization opportunities and ensuring compliance with coding guidelines.

Conclusion

The DRG system plays a critical role in the reimbursement process for inpatient hospital services, directly affecting the financial health of healthcare institutions. By focusing on accurate documentation, effective CDI programs, and continuous staff education, healthcare providers can navigate the complexities of DRG assignment, ensuring fair and adequate reimbursement for the services they provide.

12.4. Inpatient vs. Outpatient Coding

Inpatient and outpatient coding are foundational elements of medical billing and coding, each with its specific guidelines and nuances. Understanding the differences between these two coding environments is crucial for coders, as it affects how services are documented, coded, and reimbursed. This comparison highlights the key distinctions and shared challenges between inpatient and outpatient coding practices.

Key Differences

1. Setting and Duration of Care:

- **Inpatient care** involves treatment where the patient is formally admitted to a healthcare facility with the expectation of staying at least one night.

- **Outpatient care** includes services where the patient receives care or undergoes procedures but does not stay overnight.

2. Coding Systems Used:

- **Inpatient coding** primarily utilizes ICD-10-CM for diagnoses and ICD-10-PCS for procedures.

- **Outpatient coding** employs ICD-10-CM for diagnoses, CPT (Current Procedural Terminology) for procedures and services, and HCPCS Level II for additional supplies, drugs, and durable medical equipment.

3. Focus of Coding:

- Inpatient coding focuses on capturing the patient's entire encounter from admission to discharge, emphasizing conditions that affect the patient's stay and treatment.

- Outpatient coding centers on the specific services provided during the visit, with a strong emphasis on procedural coding.

4. Reimbursement Methodologies:

- **Inpatient services** are typically reimbursed based on Diagnosis-Related Groups (DRGs), which consider the patient's condition, procedures performed, and other factors.

- **Outpatient services** are generally reimbursed per procedure or service, often guided by fee schedules or negotiated rates.

Shared Challenges

Despite their differences, both inpatient and outpatient coding face common challenges, including:

- **Keeping Up with Coding Updates:** Both areas require coders to stay current with changes in coding guidelines, new codes, and deleted codes across ICD-10-CM, ICD-10-PCS, CPT, and HCPCS Level II.

- **Documentation Quality:** Accurate and complete documentation from healthcare providers is vital for correct code assignment in both settings.

- **Compliance and Accuracy:** Ensuring coding practices comply with regulatory standards and accurately reflect the care provided is a constant concern to avoid audits and claim denials.

Strategies for Success in Both Settings

- **Continuous Education and Training:** Coders should engage in ongoing education to keep abreast of the latest coding standards and best practices for both inpatient and outpatient settings.

- **Quality Assurance Processes:** Implementing regular audits and feedback mechanisms can help identify and correct coding inaccuracies and improve documentation practices.

- **Collaboration with Healthcare Providers:** Effective communication between coders and healthcare providers is essential for clarifying documentation and ensuring accurate coding.

- **Leveraging Technology:** Utilizing advanced coding software and electronic health record (EHR) systems can enhance coding accuracy and efficiency.

Conclusion

While inpatient and outpatient coding serve different facets of healthcare services, both are integral to the healthcare revenue cycle management. By understanding the distinctions and embracing strategies to address shared challenges, coders can ensure accuracy, compliance, and optimal reimbursement across both inpatient and outpatient settings.

12.5. Exercise: 10 MCQs with Answers at the End

Test your knowledge on Specialty Coding II: Inpatient Services, including the basics of inpatient coding, coding for complex inpatient cases, DRGs, and the differences between inpatient and outpatient coding. Answers are provided at the end for self-assessment.

Questions

1. Which coding system is used for inpatient procedure coding?

   A. CPT

   B. ICD-10-CM

   C. ICD-10-PCS

   D. HCPCS Level II

2. The primary diagnosis in inpatient coding is defined as:

   A. The most expensive diagnosis to treat

   B. The diagnosis that requires the most extended stay

   C. The condition established after study to be chiefly responsible for the hospital admission

   D. Any chronic condition the patient has

3. Diagnosis-Related Groups (DRGs) are used primarily for:

A. Outpatient procedure coding

B. Determining physician fees

C. Inpatient hospital reimbursement

D. Classifying medications

4. What is a major challenge in inpatient coding?

A. The simplicity of the cases

B. The high volume of outpatient cases

C. Keeping up with changes in ICD-10-PCS codes

D. The lack of need for documentation

5. What differentiates inpatient from outpatient coding in terms of reimbursement methodology?

A. Inpatient services are reimbursed per service

B. Outpatient services use DRGs for reimbursement

C. Inpatient services are typically reimbursed based on DRGs

D. There is no difference in reimbursement methods

6. A Clinical Documentation Improvement (CDI) program is essential for:

A. Reducing the length of patient stays

B. Improving the accuracy of clinical documentation for coding purposes

C. Eliminating the need for coders

D. Increasing the number of outpatient procedures

7. In outpatient coding, which codes are primarily used for procedures?

A. ICD-10-CM

B. CPT

C. ICD-10-PCS

D. DRGs

8. Secondary diagnoses in inpatient coding:

A. Have no impact on DRG assignment

B. Are ignored if they don't require treatment

C. Can affect the severity level and DRG assignment

D. Are only coded if they are related to the principal diagnosis

9. A key strategy to optimize DRG assignment and reimbursement is:

 A. Assigning the DRG with the highest reimbursement regardless of accuracy

 B. Implementing robust Clinical Documentation Improvement (CDI) programs

 C. Avoiding coding secondary diagnoses

 D. Using outpatient codes for inpatient services

10. Which is true about the ICD-10-PCS coding system?

 A. It is used for both inpatient and outpatient procedure coding

 B. It provides a high level of specificity for inpatient procedures

 C. It is the primary system for coding diagnoses in outpatient settings

 D. It replaces CPT codes in outpatient settings

Answers

1. C. ICD-10-PCS

2. C. The condition established after study to be chiefly responsible for the hospital admission

3. C. Inpatient hospital reimbursement

4. C. Keeping up with changes in ICD-10-PCS codes

5. C. Inpatient services are typically reimbursed based on DRGs

6. B. Improving the accuracy of clinical documentation for coding purposes

7. B. CPT

8. C. Can affect the severity level and DRG assignment

9. B. Implementing robust Clinical Documentation Improvement (CDI) programs

10. B. It provides a high level of specificity for inpatient procedures

These questions and answers aim to reinforce key concepts related to inpatient services coding, highlighting the distinct coding systems, the role of DRGs in reimbursement, and the importance of accurate documentation and coding practices.

Chapter 13: Specialty Coding III: Emergency Medicine

13.1. Emergency Department Coding Basics

Emergency department (ED) coding involves documenting and coding the medical care and services provided to patients in the emergency department. This unique coding specialty requires a thorough understanding of the coding guidelines specific to emergency medicine, which can differ significantly from those in other healthcare settings due to the urgent and varied nature of emergency care.

Key Aspects of Emergency Department Coding

1. CPT Codes for Services and Procedures:

- Emergency department coding primarily uses Current Procedural Terminology (CPT) codes to document the wide range of services and procedures provided, from initial assessments to complex interventions.

2. ICD-10-CM Codes for Diagnoses:

- Diagnoses are coded using the International Classification of Diseases, Tenth Revision, Clinical Modification (ICD-10-CM), focusing on the condition that necessitated the emergency visit.

3. Facility vs. Professional Coding:

- ED coding includes both facility coding (for the use of emergency department resources) and professional coding (for the medical services provided by physicians and other healthcare professionals).

4. Use of E/M (Evaluation and Management) Codes:

- E/M codes are frequently used in ED coding to capture the level of care and complexity of patient evaluations. The selection of the appropriate E/M code is based on factors such as the patient's history, examination, and medical decision-making complexity.

Challenges in Emergency Department Coding

1. Variability of Cases:

- Emergency departments treat a wide range of conditions, from minor injuries to life-threatening emergencies, making coding for these services complex and varied.

2. Documentation Quality:

- Accurate and complete documentation is crucial for proper coding but can be challenging to obtain in the fast-paced, high-stress environment of the emergency department.

3. Determining the Level of E/M Services:

- Selecting the correct level of E/M service requires careful consideration of the documentation, which can be subjective and prone to interpretation.

4. Critical Care Coding:

- Coding for critical care services involves specific criteria and time thresholds, necessitating precise documentation and coding expertise.

Strategies for Effective Emergency Department Coding

1. Continuous Education and Training:

- Coders specializing in emergency medicine should engage in ongoing education to stay current with coding guidelines, especially changes to E/M coding and critical care criteria.

2. Close Collaboration with Healthcare Providers:

- Working closely with ED physicians and staff to improve documentation practices can significantly enhance coding accuracy and compliance.

3. Utilize Coding Resources and Tools:

- Access to up-to-date coding manuals, online resources, and coding software can aid in accurate code selection and verification.

4. Implement Quality Assurance Measures:

- Regular audits and quality checks of coded data can identify patterns of errors or inconsistencies, allowing for timely corrections and feedback to coding staff and healthcare providers.

Conclusion

Emergency department coding is a critical component of healthcare coding, requiring a unique set of skills and knowledge due to the urgent and diverse nature of emergency care. By focusing on accurate documentation, continuous education, and effective collaboration between coders and healthcare providers, coding professionals can navigate the challenges of ED coding, ensuring appropriate reimbursement and compliance with coding standards.

13.2. Coding for Trauma and Acute Care

Coding for trauma and acute care presents unique challenges due to the urgent and complex nature of these services. Trauma coding involves documenting emergency care provided to patients with life-threatening or potentially disabling injuries. Acute care coding covers a broad range of intensive, immediate treatments given in emergency departments (EDs), trauma centers, and critical care units. Accuracy in coding these encounters is critical for ensuring proper reimbursement, facilitating quality patient care, and contributing to trauma registries and public health data.

Key Considerations in Trauma and Acute Care Coding

1. Comprehensive Documentation:

- Detailed documentation is essential to capture the full scope of care provided to trauma and acute care patients, including the extent of injuries, all procedures performed, and the critical care services rendered.

2. ICD-10-CM Injury Codes:

- Accurate assignment of ICD-10-CM codes for injuries, including external cause codes, is crucial for trauma coding. These codes provide valuable data for injury research and prevention strategies.

3. CPT and HCPCS Codes for Procedures:

- Utilizing Current Procedural Terminology (CPT) and Healthcare Common Procedure Coding System (HCPCS) codes accurately reflects the surgical procedures, emergency services, and other treatments provided to patients.

4. Critical Care Services:

- Coding for critical care services requires identifying when patients receive continuous, direct care for life-threatening conditions. Documentation should support the amount of time spent on critical care, which directly impacts coding and billing.

Challenges in Coding for Trauma and Acute Care

1. High-Stress, Fast-Paced Environment:

- The urgency associated with trauma and acute care can impact the completeness and clarity of documentation, posing challenges for coders trying to accurately code these services.

2. Multidisciplinary Care:

- Patients often receive care from multiple specialists, necessitating a coordinated approach to documentation and coding to capture all aspects of care accurately.

3. Severity and Complexity of Cases:

- Trauma and acute care cases often involve severe, complex injuries requiring detailed coding to capture the full extent of care provided and resources utilized.

4. External Cause Codes:

- Determining the appropriate external cause codes (e.g., codes for accidents, violence) can be complex but is essential for trauma registries and epidemiological studies.

Strategies for Effective Coding in Trauma and Acute Care

1. Specialized Training:

- Coders specializing in trauma and acute care should receive targeted training in trauma anatomy, emergency medicine procedures, and the specific coding guidelines applicable to trauma and critical care.

2. Close Collaboration with Clinical Staff:

- Building strong communication channels with physicians, nurses, and other healthcare providers ensures that coders have access to comprehensive and accurate documentation.

3. Use of Trauma Registries:

- Participating in or accessing trauma registries can enhance the accuracy of coding by providing additional insights into common trauma cases and coding practices.

4. Regular Audits and Feedback:

- Conducting regular coding audits and providing feedback to both coders and clinical staff can help identify areas for improvement, ensuring more accurate and comprehensive coding over time.

Conclusion

Coding for trauma and acute care is an intricate process that requires specialized knowledge, attention to detail, and effective communication with clinical teams. By addressing the unique challenges of these high-stress environments and employing strategic approaches to documentation and coding, healthcare organizations can ensure accurate coding practices, supporting optimal patient care and appropriate reimbursement.

13.3. E/M Coding in Emergency Medicine

Evaluation and Management (E/M) coding in emergency medicine is a critical aspect of medical billing that reflects the complexity and intensity of care provided to patients in emergency settings. E/M codes are used to document the level of medical decision-making, the time spent with the patient, and the nature of the presenting problem. Proper use of E/M codes in emergency medicine is essential for accurate reimbursement, compliance with coding standards, and effective communication of patient care efforts.

Key Components of E/M Coding in Emergency Medicine

1. Levels of E/M Services:

- E/M services in emergency medicine are categorized into different levels based on the complexity of medical decision-making, the amount of time spent on patient care, and the severity of the presenting problem.

2. Three Key Components for E/M Level Selection:

  - **History:** The breadth of patient history obtained, including history of present illness, review of systems, and past/family/social history.

  - **Examination:** The extent of the physical exam conducted on the patient.

  - **Medical Decision Making (MDM):** The complexity of establishing diagnoses, analyzing test results, and formulating a treatment plan.

3. Time-Based Coding:

- For cases where time is the primary factor, such as in critical care, E/M codes may be selected based on the total time spent providing direct care to the patient during the emergency department visit.

Challenges in E/M Coding in Emergency Medicine

1. Documentation Requirements:

- Accurate and detailed documentation is essential for substantiating the level of E/M services claimed. Inadequate documentation can lead to downcoding or denial of claims.

2. Determining the Correct Level of Care:

- Assigning the appropriate E/M level requires a nuanced understanding of the guidelines, which can be challenging given the variable nature of emergency department visits.

3. Critical Care Services:

- Identifying when a patient's condition warrants critical care services and documenting the time spent in critical care can be complex, requiring careful attention to coding rules.

Strategies for Effective E/M Coding in Emergency Medicine

1. Regular Training and Education:

- Coders and healthcare providers should engage in continuous education on the latest E/M coding guidelines, including any updates specific to emergency medicine.

2. Comprehensive Documentation:

- Encourage healthcare providers to document thoroughly, covering all aspects of patient history, examination findings, and the rationale for medical decision-making.

3. Utilize Coding Tools and Resources:

- Leveraging coding software and resources that provide guidance on E/M coding can help coders accurately determine the appropriate level of service.

4. Collaboration Between Coders and Clinicians:

- Foster open communication between clinical staff and coders to clarify documentation and ensure the accurate reflection of the care provided.

5. Conduct Regular Audits:

- Implementing a system for regular audits of E/M coding can identify patterns of errors or discrepancies and provide opportunities for feedback and improvement.

Conclusion

E/M coding in emergency medicine is a complex process that plays a vital role in the reimbursement cycle and the overall documentation of patient care. By addressing the challenges associated with E/M coding through education, thorough documentation, and collaboration, healthcare providers can ensure accurate and compliant coding practices that reflect the level of care provided in emergency settings.

13.4. Challenges in Emergency Medicine Coding

Coding in emergency medicine presents unique challenges due to the unpredictable nature of the cases, the urgency of care required, and the complexity of documenting such encounters accurately. Emergency department (ED) coders must navigate these challenges to ensure precise coding, which is crucial for appropriate reimbursement, compliance with healthcare regulations, and the accurate representation of patient care.

Key Challenges in Emergency Medicine Coding

1. Rapid and Varied Patient Care:

- The ED handles a wide range of conditions, from minor injuries to life-threatening emergencies. Coders must be proficient in a broad spectrum of medical terminology and coding guidelines to accurately capture the diversity of care provided.

2. Documentation Quality and Completeness:

- High patient volumes and the fast-paced environment can lead to incomplete or nonspecific documentation, making it difficult for coders to determine the correct codes.

3. Critical Care Coding:

- Identifying and coding for critical care services require understanding specific criteria, such as time spent on direct patient care. Documenting and coding these services accurately can be challenging.

4. Use of E/M Codes:

- Determining the appropriate level of Evaluation and Management (E/M) services based on documentation can be subjective, leading to variability in coding practices.

5. Modifier Application:

- Correctly applying modifiers to indicate specific circumstances of the care provided (e.g., procedures performed during the ED visit) is essential but can be complex.

6. Compliance with Coding Guidelines:

- Emergency medicine coding must adhere to various coding guidelines and payer-specific rules, which are subject to change, adding another layer of complexity.

Strategies to Address These Challenges

1. Continuous Education and Training:

- Providing ongoing education for coders on the latest coding guidelines, medical terminology, and emergency medicine practices is essential to keep skills current.

2. Enhancing Documentation Practices:

- Collaborating with clinicians to improve the quality of medical documentation in the ED can significantly aid coding accuracy. Implementing structured documentation templates may help.

3. Utilizing Technology:

- Advanced coding software and electronic health records (EHRs) with built-in prompts and checks can assist coders in capturing all necessary information for accurate coding.

4. Regular Audits and Quality Checks:

- Conducting periodic coding audits can identify common errors or discrepancies, offering opportunities for feedback and improvement.

5. Clear Communication Channels:

- Establishing effective communication channels between coders and clinicians allows for timely clarification of documentation, enhancing coding accuracy.

6. Emphasizing the Importance of Modifier Use:

- Providing specific training on the correct application of modifiers in emergency medicine coding can reduce errors and ensure compliance.

Conclusion

The challenges in emergency medicine coding are significant, stemming from the unique nature of emergency care. However, with targeted strategies such as continuous education, improved documentation practices, and the use of technology, coders can overcome these obstacles. By doing so, they ensure that coding accurately reflects the care provided, supporting optimal reimbursement and compliance with healthcare regulations.

13.5. Exercise: 10 MCQs with Answers at the End

Test your knowledge on Specialty Coding III: Emergency Medicine, including the basics of emergency department coding, coding for trauma and acute care, E/M coding in emergency medicine, and challenges specific to emergency medicine coding. Answers are provided at the end for self-assessment.

Questions

1. Which coding system is primarily used for documenting procedures in the emergency department?

A. ICD-10-CM

B. CPT

C. ICD-10-PCS

D. HCPCS Level II

2. What is essential for accurately coding emergency department visits?

A. The patient's insurance information

B. Comprehensive documentation of the visit

C. The number of patients waiting in the ED

D. The time of day the patient arrives

3. Which of the following best describes E/M coding in emergency medicine?

A. It's based solely on the patient's diagnosis.

B. It determines the facility's cleanliness.

C. It reflects the complexity and intensity of evaluating and managing the patient.

D. It's used to code only surgical procedures.

4. Critical care coding in emergency medicine is determined by:

A. The age of the patient

B. The total time spent on direct care for a critically ill or critically injured patient

C. The number of tests ordered

D. The patient's ability to pay

5. Challenges in emergency medicine coding include:

A. Too few codes to cover all possible scenarios

B. Rapid and varied patient care

C. The predictability of cases

D. Lower patient volumes compared to other departments

6. A key strategy to address challenges in emergency medicine coding is:

A. Decreasing documentation requirements

B. Using only generic codes for all ED visits

C. Continuous education and training

D. Avoiding the use of E/M codes

7. In emergency medicine coding, modifiers are used to indicate:

   A. Only services provided by the head nurse

   B. Specific circumstances surrounding a procedure

   C. The emergency department's location within the hospital

   D. The patient's discharge instructions

8. The correct application of E/M codes in the ED depends on:

   A. The patient's previous medical history

   B. Documentation covering the history, examination, and medical decision-making

   C. The color of the patient's wristband

   D. Whether the patient is a minor

9. Which document is crucial for coding trauma and acute care cases accurately?

   A. The hospital's annual report

   B. The detailed surgical report and physician's notes

   C. The cafeteria menu for the day of the visit

   D. The insurance claim form completed by the patient

10. Effective communication between coders and clinicians in the ED is important for:

    A. Deciding who takes the lunch break first

    B. Ensuring accurate and complete documentation for coding

    C. Discussing personal plans for the weekend

    D. Choosing the color scheme for the ED

Answers

1. B. CPT

2. B. Comprehensive documentation of the visit

3. C. It reflects the complexity and intensity of evaluating and managing the patient.

4. B. The total time spent on direct care for a critically ill or critically injured patient

5. B. Rapid and varied patient care

6. C. Continuous education and training

7. B. Specific circumstances surrounding a procedure

8. B. Documentation covering the history, examination, and medical decision-making

9. B. The detailed surgical report and physician's notes

10. B. Ensuring accurate and complete documentation for coding

Chapter 14: Specialty Coding IV: Obstetrics and Gynecology

14.1. OB/GYN Coding Overview

Obstetrics and Gynecology (OB/GYN) coding encompasses the documentation and coding of services related to women's health, including pregnancy, childbirth, and the reproductive system. Coding in OB/GYN requires a deep understanding of specific coding guidelines, as well as the ability to navigate the complexities associated with procedures, treatments, and conditions unique to this specialty.

Key Aspects of OB/GYN Coding

1. CPT Codes for Procedures and Services:

- OB/GYN coding utilizes Current Procedural Terminology (CPT) codes to document surgical procedures, office visits, obstetric care, and other gynecological services.

2. ICD-10-CM Codes for Diagnoses:

- Diagnoses are coded using the International Classification of Diseases, Tenth Revision, Clinical Modification (ICD-10-CM), focusing on conditions specific to obstetrics and gynecology, such as pregnancy complications, menstrual disorders, and other reproductive system conditions.

3. Global Obstetric (OB) Care:

- Global OB care coding covers the comprehensive care provided throughout pregnancy, delivery, and the postpartum period, typically bundled into a single code that encompasses prenatal visits, delivery, and postnatal care.

4. Use of Modifiers:

- Modifiers are essential in OB/GYN coding to indicate specific circumstances, such as when only part of the global OB care package is provided or when complications require additional services.

Challenges in OB/GYN Coding

1. Understanding Global OB Care Packages:

- Coders must accurately determine what services are included in the global care package and identify when separate billing for additional procedures or complications is justified.

2. Documentation and Specificity:

- Detailed and specific documentation is crucial, especially for conditions that have a significant impact on the type of care provided, such as high-risk pregnancies.

3. Coding for Multiple Gestations:

- Pregnancies involving twins, triplets, or more present coding challenges, requiring coders to document each fetus's care accurately.

4. Keeping Up with Coding Updates:

- OB/GYN coding guidelines and codes, particularly those related to new procedures and technologies, are regularly updated, necessitating continuous education.

Strategies for Effective OB/GYN Coding

1. Continuous Education and Training:

- Coders specializing in OB/GYN should engage in ongoing education to stay abreast of the latest coding guidelines, CPT updates, and ICD-10-CM changes.

2. Comprehensive Documentation Review:

- Thoroughly review medical records for complete documentation that supports coding decisions, especially for procedures outside the global OB package or for conditions affecting pregnancy and delivery.

3. Collaboration with Healthcare Providers:

- Work closely with OB/GYN practitioners to ensure accurate and detailed documentation, facilitating appropriate code assignment and reimbursement.

4. Utilization of Coding Resources and Tools:

- Leverage coding manuals, online resources, and professional coding forums specific to OB/GYN to resolve coding questions and ensure accurate code selection.

Conclusion

OB/GYN coding is a specialized area that requires coders to have a detailed understanding of the comprehensive care associated with obstetrics and gynecology. By mastering the complexities of coding for this specialty, coders can ensure accurate billing and support the financial health of healthcare providers, while also contributing to the delivery of quality care to patients.

14.2. Coding for Obstetric Procedures

Coding for obstetric (OB) procedures involves documenting the range of medical services provided to women during pregnancy, labor, delivery, and the postpartum period. It requires a specialized understanding of the obstetric care continuum, from prenatal visits to postnatal care, and the ability to accurately apply codes that reflect the complexity and nature of each service.

Key Components in Coding Obstetric Procedures

1. Global Obstetric Package:

- The global OB package encompasses comprehensive care for the expectant mother, including prenatal visits, labor and delivery, and postpartum care. It is typically coded with a single CPT code that covers the entire continuum of care, assuming a normal, uncomplicated pregnancy.

2. Prenatal and Postnatal Visits:

- Routine prenatal and postnatal care visits are included in the global package. However, any services outside the standard care—for example, treatment for complications or additional diagnostic testing—may need to be coded separately.

3. Labor and Delivery:

- Coding for labor and delivery must accurately reflect the method of delivery (e.g., vaginal, cesarean section, VBAC— vaginal birth after cesarean), any complications encountered, and whether the delivery involved twins or higher-order multiples.

4. Complications of Pregnancy:

- Complications such as gestational diabetes, preeclampsia, or preterm labor require additional coding to document the complexity of care provided. ICD-10-CM codes offer specific options for detailing these conditions.

5. Procedures Beyond Global Package:

- Certain obstetric procedures fall outside the global package and need separate coding. These can include specialized ultrasounds, fetal non-stress tests, and amniocentesis.

Challenges in Coding Obstetric Procedures

1. Determining Global Package Components:

- Understanding what is included in the global OB package and identifying services that warrant separate billing can be challenging.

2. Documentation Accuracy:

- Detailed and clear documentation is crucial for supporting the codes selected, especially for complications or additional procedures not covered by the global package.

3. Multiple Gestations:

- Coding for pregnancies involving twins or more requires specific attention to detail to ensure each fetus's care is accurately documented and billed.

4. Staying Updated with Guidelines:

- Obstetric coding guidelines and codes are subject to change, making it essential for coders to stay informed about the latest updates.

Strategies for Effective Obstetric Coding

1. Continuous Education:

- Regular training on current OB coding practices, guidelines, and updates is vital for maintaining accuracy and compliance.

2. Thorough Documentation Review:

- Carefully review all documentation related to prenatal visits, labor and delivery, and postpartum care to ensure comprehensive coding.

3. Clear Communication with Healthcare Providers:

- Establish effective communication channels with OB/GYN practitioners to clarify documentation, especially for complicated cases or when services extend beyond the global package.

4. Utilize Coding Resources:

- Make use of professional coding manuals, online resources, and coding forums specific to OB/GYN to resolve complex coding issues and ensure accurate code selection.

Conclusion

Coding for obstetric procedures is a complex but critical component of medical coding in the field of OB/GYN. By applying a deep understanding of the obstetric care continuum, staying informed about coding updates, and ensuring accurate documentation, coders can effectively navigate the intricacies of obstetric coding. This ensures appropriate reimbursement for healthcare providers and contributes to the overall quality of care for expectant mothers.

14.3. Gynecological Surgery Coding

Gynecological surgery coding involves documenting surgical procedures related to the female reproductive system, excluding those directly associated with childbirth. This specialized area of coding requires an in-depth understanding of the procedures, the anatomy of the female reproductive system, and the specific coding guidelines applicable to gynecological surgeries.

Key Aspects of Gynecological Surgery Coding

1. CPT Codes for Surgical Procedures:

- Gynecological surgeries are primarily coded using Current Procedural Terminology (CPT) codes. These codes cover a wide range of procedures, from minor office-based surgeries to major operations.

2. ICD-10-CM Codes for Diagnoses:

- Accurate diagnosis coding using ICD-10-CM is essential to establish the medical necessity of the surgical procedure and to support the use of specific CPT codes.

3. Use of Modifiers:

- Modifiers play a crucial role in gynecological surgery coding, indicating circumstances such as surgeries performed on both sides of the body (bilateral), multiple procedures, or services that are distinct from those normally performed together.

4. Documentation Requirements:

- Detailed surgical reports and physician documentation are vital for accurate coding. Documentation should clearly describe the procedure, findings, and any complications encountered.

Challenges in Gynecological Surgery Coding

1. Complexity of Procedures:

- Gynecological surgeries can range from straightforward to highly complex, involving advanced techniques and technologies. Understanding the nuances of each procedure is critical for accurate coding.

2. Keeping Up with Advances in Surgical Techniques:

- As new surgical technologies and techniques are developed, such as robotic-assisted surgery, coders must stay informed to code these procedures accurately.

3. Differentiating Similar Procedures:

- Some gynecological procedures are very similar but have distinct codes. Coders must carefully differentiate between these procedures based on the specifics documented in the surgical report.

4. Identifying Complications and Comorbidities:

- Coding for complications or coexisting conditions requires a thorough review of the patient's medical record to ensure comprehensive and accurate coding.

Strategies for Effective Gynecological Surgery Coding

1. Continuous Education and Training:

- Regular participation in coding education and training programs specific to gynecology can help coders stay current with coding guidelines, surgical techniques, and technology advancements.

2. Utilize Specialty-Specific Coding Resources:

- Access to gynecology-specific coding manuals, guidelines, and online resources can aid in accurate code selection and staying updated on coding changes.

3. Collaborate with Healthcare Providers:

- Effective communication with surgeons and other healthcare providers is essential for clarifying procedure details, ensuring documentation completeness, and resolving coding queries.

4. Perform Regular Coding Audits:

- Conducting periodic audits of gynecological surgery coding can identify areas for improvement, reduce coding errors, and enhance compliance with coding standards.

Conclusion

Gynecological surgery coding is a specialized field that demands a detailed understanding of surgical procedures, anatomy, and coding guidelines. By embracing continuous education, utilizing specialized resources, and fostering collaboration with healthcare providers, coders can navigate the complexities of this area, ensuring accurate and compliant coding practices. This not only supports proper reimbursement but also contributes to the quality of patient care in the field of gynecology.

14.4. Coding for Maternal and Fetal Complications

Coding for maternal and fetal complications involves documenting various conditions that can occur during pregnancy, labor, and delivery, which may adversely affect the health of the mother, the fetus, or both. Accurate coding of these complications is critical for ensuring appropriate care management, supporting research on maternal and fetal health, and securing accurate reimbursement for healthcare services.

Key Considerations in Coding for Maternal and Fetal Complications

1. ICD-10-CM Codes:

- Maternal and fetal complications are primarily coded using the International Classification of Diseases, Tenth Revision, Clinical Modification (ICD-10-CM). This system provides detailed codes that describe specific complications and conditions.

2. Specificity and Detail:

- The specificity of the coding is paramount. Codes are available to represent the trimester of pregnancy during which the complication occurred, the specific type of complication, and whether the complication is related to the current pregnancy or a previous one.

3. Linking Conditions to Pregnancy:

- It's important to clearly link the complication to the pregnancy in the coding process. This ensures that the complication is recognized as a factor influencing patient care and outcomes during the pregnancy.

4. Sequencing of Codes:

- Proper sequencing of codes is crucial, especially when coding for multiple complications. The principal diagnosis is typically the condition most responsible for the hospital admission or care provided.

Challenges in Coding for Maternal and Fetal Complications

1. Documentation Quality:

- Inadequate or nonspecific documentation can significantly hinder the ability to accurately code complications, requiring coders to seek additional information from healthcare providers.

2. Complex Clinical Scenarios:

- Pregnancies with multiple complications present a coding challenge, as coders must navigate complex clinical information to accurately document all relevant conditions.

3. Keeping Up with Guidelines:

- Coding guidelines for obstetrics, particularly those related to complications, are subject to change. Staying current with these guidelines is essential for accurate coding.

4. Differentiating Between Conditions:

- Some maternal and fetal conditions have similar clinical features or names but are coded differently. Distinguishing between these conditions requires a deep understanding of obstetric medical terminology and coding guidelines.

Strategies for Effective Coding of Maternal and Fetal Complications

1. Continuous Education and Training:

- Coders should engage in ongoing education focused on obstetric coding, including the coding of complications, to stay informed about the latest coding practices and guidelines.

2. Thorough Documentation Review:

- Carefully review all available documentation, including physician notes, laboratory results, and imaging studies, to ensure a comprehensive understanding of the patient's condition and the complications present.

3. Collaboration with Healthcare Providers:

- Establishing strong communication channels with obstetricians and other healthcare providers is crucial for clarifying documentation and ensuring that all relevant complications are accurately coded.

4. Utilization of Coding Resources:

- Access to up-to-date coding manuals, online resources, and professional coding forums can provide valuable assistance in coding complex maternal and fetal complications.

Conclusion

Coding for maternal and fetal complications requires a nuanced approach to accurately capture the complexity of obstetric care. By employing strategies such as continuous education, thorough documentation review, and collaboration with healthcare providers, coders can effectively navigate the challenges associated with documenting these conditions. This not only supports appropriate billing and reimbursement but also contributes to the overall quality of maternal and fetal healthcare.

14.5. Exercise: 10 MCQs with Answers at the End

Test your understanding of Specialty Coding IV: Obstetrics and Gynecology, covering OB/GYN coding overview, coding for obstetric procedures, gynecological surgery coding, coding for maternal and fetal complications, and associated challenges. Answers are provided at the end for self-assessment.

Questions

1. What coding system is primarily used for gynecological surgery procedures?

   A. ICD-10-CM

   B. CPT

   C. ICD-10-PCS

D. HCPCS Level II

2. The global OB care package includes all of the following EXCEPT:

A. Prenatal visits

B. Delivery

C. Postpartum care

D. Treatment for unrelated chronic conditions

3. Which of the following is essential for coding maternal and fetal complications accurately?

A. Specifying the trimester in which the complication occurred

B. Coding all pregnancies as high-risk

C. Using only general codes for pregnancy complications

D. Ignoring fetal conditions if the mother is healthy

4. Modifiers in OB/GYN coding are used to indicate:

A. The gender of the baby

B. Specific circumstances surrounding a procedure

C. The number of babies delivered

D. The marital status of the mother

5. Challenges in OB/GYN coding do NOT include:

A. High patient volume

B. Complex clinical scenarios

C. Frequent changes in non-OB/GYN coding guidelines

D. Documentation quality

6. Critical care coding in emergency medicine for obstetric cases is determined by:

A. The patient's age

B. The total time spent on direct care for a critically ill patient

C. The number of doctors present

D. The patient's insurance coverage

7. Effective strategies for coding in OB/GYN include all EXCEPT:

A. Decreasing communication with healthcare providers

B. Continuous education and training

C. Utilization of coding resources

D. Regular audits and quality checks

8. In gynecological surgery coding, the use of ICD-10-PCS codes is for:

A. Documenting procedures in outpatient settings

B. Coding the diagnoses related to the surgeries

C. Documenting procedures in inpatient settings

D. Coding the length of hospital stay

9. Coding for obstetric procedures must accurately reflect:

A. Only the method of delivery

B. The method of delivery, complications encountered, and care provided

C. The preferred names for the newborns

D. The time of day the delivery occurred

10. A major challenge in coding for maternal and fetal complications is:

A. The simplicity of the cases

B. Distinguishing between similar conditions with different codes

C. Coding only in the first trimester

D. Avoiding the use of ICD-10-CM codes

Answers

1. B. CPT

2. D. Treatment for unrelated chronic conditions

3. A. Specifying the trimester in which the complication occurred

4. B. Specific circumstances surrounding a procedure

5. C. Frequent changes in non-OB/GYN coding guidelines

6. B. The total time spent on direct care for a critically ill patient

7. A. Decreasing communication with healthcare providers

8. C. Documenting procedures in inpatient settings

9. B. The method of delivery, complications encountered, and care provided

10. B. Distinguishing between similar conditions with different codes

These questions and answers aim to reinforce key concepts in OB/GYN coding, emphasizing the importance of accurate documentation, continuous education, and effective strategies to address coding challenges in obstetrics and gynecology.

Chapter 15: Specialty Coding V: Pediatrics

15.1. Pediatric Coding Basics

Pediatric coding encompasses the documentation and coding of medical services provided to infants, children, and adolescents. Given the unique healthcare needs of this population, pediatric coding requires a thorough understanding of the growth and development stages, common pediatric illnesses and conditions, and preventive care measures. Accurate coding in pediatrics is crucial for ensuring proper reimbursement, facilitating patient care management, and contributing to pediatric healthcare research and policy development.

Key Aspects of Pediatric Coding

1. ICD-10-CM Codes for Diagnoses:

- Diagnoses in pediatric coding are documented using the International Classification of Diseases, Tenth Revision, Clinical Modification (ICD-10-CM). Coders must be familiar with codes specific to pediatric conditions and developmental stages.

2. CPT Codes for Procedures and Services:

- Current Procedural Terminology (CPT) codes are used to document procedures, treatments, and other healthcare services provided to pediatric patients. This includes routine immunizations, developmental screenings, and surgical procedures.

3. Preventive Care and Well-Child Visits:

- Pediatric coding often involves preventive care services, such as well-child visits, which are coded differently from illness or condition-specific visits. Understanding the coding guidelines for preventive services is essential.

4. Age-Specific Coding Considerations:

- Certain codes and guidelines are specific to the patient's age, reflecting the unique healthcare needs at different stages of childhood and adolescence.

Challenges in Pediatric Coding

1. Documentation Quality:

- Adequate and specific documentation is vital for accurate pediatric coding. Documentation must clearly detail the reason for the visit, findings, and any treatments provided.

2. Coding for Chronic Conditions and Comorbidities:

- Many pediatric patients have chronic conditions (e.g., asthma, diabetes) that require ongoing management. Coding these conditions alongside acute illnesses or conditions can be complex.

3. Immunization Coding:

- Immunizations are a significant part of pediatric care. Coding for vaccines involves not only the administration codes but also the specific vaccine product codes, which can be numerous and frequently updated.

4. Preventive Services Guidelines:

- Coding guidelines for preventive services, such as well-child visits, are periodically updated. Staying informed about these changes is crucial for pediatric coders.

Strategies for Effective Pediatric Coding

1. Continuous Education and Training:

- Pediatric coders should engage in ongoing education to stay current with the latest ICD-10-CM and CPT coding updates, particularly those relevant to pediatrics.

2. Thorough Documentation Review:

- Carefully reviewing medical records for complete and specific documentation supports accurate coding and helps identify any services that may require additional clarification from healthcare providers.

3. Use of Pediatric Coding Resources:

- Utilizing coding resources and tools specific to pediatrics, including pediatric coding manuals and online forums, can aid in resolving coding queries and challenges.

4. Collaboration with Healthcare Providers:

- Effective communication and collaboration with pediatricians and other healthcare providers are essential for clarifying documentation and ensuring that all services are accurately coded.

Conclusion

Pediatric coding plays a vital role in the healthcare billing process, requiring a specialized understanding of pediatric healthcare services and coding guidelines. By addressing the unique challenges of pediatric coding through continuous education, thorough documentation review, and collaboration with healthcare providers, coders can ensure accurate and compliant coding practices. This not only supports the financial health of healthcare organizations but also contributes to the overall quality of pediatric healthcare.

15.2. Coding for Common Pediatric Conditions

Coding for common pediatric conditions involves a nuanced understanding of the diseases and health issues that frequently affect children and adolescents. These conditions range from acute illnesses, like ear infections and strep throat, to chronic diseases, such as asthma and diabetes. Accurate coding of these conditions is crucial for effective patient care management, tracking public health trends, and ensuring appropriate reimbursement for healthcare services.

Key Considerations in Coding for Common Pediatric Conditions

1. ICD-10-CM Codes for Diagnoses:

- The International Classification of Diseases, Tenth Revision, Clinical Modification (ICD-10-CM) is used to code pediatric diagnoses. Coders must select codes that accurately reflect the condition diagnosed, considering age-specific factors and disease manifestations in children.

2. Chronic vs. Acute Conditions:

- Differentiating between chronic conditions that require ongoing management and acute illnesses is essential for coding. Chronic conditions may also affect the coding of acute episodes by providing context and indicating complexity.

3. Coding for Developmental and Behavioral Disorders:

- Pediatric coding encompasses developmental and behavioral disorders, such as autism spectrum disorders and attention-deficit/hyperactivity disorder (ADHD). These conditions require careful documentation and coding to capture the scope of care and support services provided.

4. Preventive Services and Immunizations:

- Preventive care, including well-child visits and routine immunizations, plays a significant role in pediatrics. Coding for these services involves specific codes that indicate preventive care and the administration of vaccines.

Challenges in Coding for Common Pediatric Conditions

1. Documentation Specificity:

- Detailed and specific documentation is necessary to accurately code pediatric conditions, especially for illnesses with similar symptoms or for coding complications and comorbidities.

2. Updates to Vaccine Codes:

- With frequent updates to vaccine products and immunization schedules, staying current with the correct vaccine codes and administration codes can be challenging.

3. Age-Related Coding Guidelines:

- Certain conditions and treatments are coded differently based on the patient's age, requiring coders to be aware of these guidelines to ensure accuracy.

4. Multisystem Conditions:

- Some pediatric conditions affect multiple body systems, necessitating a comprehensive coding approach to fully document the patient's healthcare needs.

Strategies for Effective Coding of Common Pediatric Conditions

1. Continuous Education and Training:

- Engaging in regular training sessions and staying updated on ICD-10-CM coding changes, especially those relevant to pediatrics, is essential for coders.

2. Utilizing Coding Resources:

- Leveraging pediatric-specific coding manuals, online resources, and professional coding forums can help address complex coding scenarios and ensure accurate code selection.

3. Collaboration with Healthcare Providers:

- Effective communication with pediatricians and other healthcare professionals is crucial for clarifying documentation and ensuring that all relevant conditions and services are accurately coded.

4. Regular Review and Auditing:

- Conducting regular reviews and audits of pediatric coding practices can help identify areas for improvement, reduce coding errors, and enhance overall coding accuracy.

Conclusion

Coding for common pediatric conditions requires a detailed understanding of the specific health issues that affect children and adolescents. By applying targeted strategies to address the unique challenges of pediatric coding, coders can ensure accurate documentation of pediatric healthcare services, contributing to the effective management of patient care and the financial stability of healthcare organizations.

15.3. Pediatric Surgery and Procedure Coding

Pediatric surgery and procedure coding involves the documentation of surgical interventions and medical procedures performed on patients from infancy through adolescence. This specialized area of coding not only requires an understanding of general coding principles but also a deep knowledge of the nuances associated with pediatric surgeries, including congenital conditions, developmental issues, and age-specific considerations.

Key Components of Pediatric Surgery and Procedure Coding

1. CPT Codes for Surgical Procedures:

- The Current Procedural Terminology (CPT) codes are utilized to document pediatric surgeries and procedures. Coders must select the codes that accurately represent the surgical interventions performed, taking into consideration the specific details and complexity of each procedure.

2. ICD-10-PCS Codes for Inpatient Procedures:

- For inpatient pediatric surgeries, the International Classification of Diseases, Tenth Revision, Procedure Coding System (ICD-10-PCS) is used. These codes provide a detailed description of the procedures, including the approach, body part, and any devices used or procedures performed.

3. ICD-10-CM Codes for Diagnoses:

- Accurate diagnosis coding using ICD-10-CM is critical for establishing the medical necessity of the surgical procedure. This includes coding for congenital conditions, injuries, or diseases that necessitate surgical intervention.

4. Use of Modifiers:

- Modifiers may be necessary to fully describe the surgical service provided, especially if the procedure deviates from the norm due to the patient's age or size, or if multiple procedures are performed during the same operative session.

Challenges in Pediatric Surgery and Procedure Coding

1. Congenital and Developmental Conditions:

- Many pediatric surgeries address congenital anomalies or developmental conditions unique to the pediatric population, requiring coders to be familiar with a wide range of conditions and their associated codes.

2. Age and Size Considerations:

- The age and physical size of pediatric patients can significantly impact the approach and techniques used in surgery, which must be accurately reflected in the coding.

3. Multidisciplinary Procedures:

- Pediatric patients often require care from multiple specialties, leading to complex surgical scenarios that involve various procedures and specialties. Coordinating and accurately coding these procedures can be challenging.

4. Documentation Quality and Specificity:

- Comprehensive and specific surgical documentation is essential for accurate coding but can be challenging to obtain. Detailed operative reports are necessary to justify the codes selected.

Strategies for Effective Pediatric Surgery and Procedure Coding

1. Specialized Training and Education:

- Coders specializing in pediatric surgery should pursue ongoing education focused on pediatric procedures, congenital conditions, and the latest coding guidelines relevant to pediatrics.

2. Utilize Pediatric-Specific Coding Resources:

- Access to pediatric surgery coding manuals, online resources, and expert forums can provide valuable assistance in navigating complex coding scenarios.

3. Collaboration with Surgical Teams:

- Establishing strong communication with pediatric surgeons and surgical teams can help clarify procedural details and ensure accurate documentation and coding.

4. Regular Review and Auditing:

- Conducting regular coding audits for pediatric surgeries can help identify coding errors, areas for improvement, and opportunities for coder education.

Conclusion

Pediatric surgery and procedure coding demand a high level of expertise and attention to detail, given the unique considerations and challenges of treating pediatric patients. By employing dedicated strategies such as specialized education, utilization of pediatric-specific resources, and collaboration with healthcare providers, coders can effectively navigate the complexities of pediatric coding, ensuring accurate documentation and appropriate reimbursement for pediatric surgical services.

15.4. Immunization and Well-Child Visit Coding

Immunization and well-child visits are fundamental components of pediatric care, focusing on preventive health measures. Accurate coding of these services is essential for documenting the delivery of care, facilitating appropriate reimbursement, and ensuring compliance with healthcare policies and guidelines.

Immunization Coding

1. CPT Codes for Vaccine Administration:

- The administration of vaccines is documented using specific CPT codes that reflect the work involved in administering the shot, including counseling patients and caregivers about the vaccine. These codes are often reported separately from the vaccine product code.

2. Vaccine Product Codes:

- Each vaccine has its associated CPT or HCPCS Level II code that represents the vaccine product itself. Coders must use the correct product code for the specific vaccine administered.

3. Use of Modifiers:

- In certain scenarios, modifiers may be necessary to accurately report immunization services, especially if multiple vaccines are administered during the same visit.

4. Documentation Requirements:

- Proper documentation must include the name of the vaccine, the date of administration, the route and site of administration, the dosage, and the name and title of the person administering the vaccine.

Well-Child Visit Coding

1. Preventive Medicine Services Codes:

- Well-child visits are coded using preventive medicine services codes in CPT, which vary based on the age of the child. These codes cover a comprehensive evaluation and preventive care services.

2. Age-Specific Guidelines:

- The selection of the correct preventive service code is crucial and should match the patient's age as well as the specific services provided during the visit, such as developmental screenings and health education.

3. Coding for Additional Services:

- If a child is diagnosed with a new or existing condition during a well-child visit, and significant additional work is required to address the condition, separate E/M codes may be billed in addition to the preventive service code, with appropriate modifiers.

Challenges in Coding for Immunization and Well-Child Visits

1. Keeping Up with Vaccine Codes:

- Vaccine product codes and administration codes can change frequently, making it challenging to stay current.

2. Distinguishing Preventive from Diagnostic Services:

- Differentiating between preventive services provided during well-child visits and additional diagnostic or treatment services that may arise during the same visit requires careful attention.

3. Documentation of Counseling and Education:

- Documenting vaccine counseling and health education provided during well-child visits is critical for supporting the use of certain codes but can often be overlooked or inadequately recorded.

Strategies for Effective Coding

1. Continuous Education and Training:

- Coders should engage in ongoing training to stay updated on the latest vaccine codes, preventive service guidelines, and coding best practices for pediatric care.

2. Utilize Coding Resources:

- Access to current coding manuals, online databases, and immunization schedules from reputable sources like the CDC can aid in accurate coding.

3. Collaborate with Healthcare Providers:

- Effective communication with pediatricians and healthcare staff ensures that all services are adequately documented and that any coding questions are promptly addressed.

4. Regular Audits and Quality Checks:

- Conducting periodic audits of immunization and well-child visit coding can help identify areas for improvement, ensuring compliance and accuracy.

Conclusion

Coding for immunizations and well-child visits requires a specialized understanding of pediatric preventive care services and attention to detail. By adopting effective coding strategies and maintaining a commitment to continuous education, coders can accurately document these essential services, supporting the health of pediatric patients and the operational success of healthcare practices.

15.5. Exercise: 10 MCQs with Answers at the End

Test your knowledge on Specialty Coding V: Pediatrics, focusing on pediatric coding basics, coding for common pediatric conditions, pediatric surgery and procedure coding, immunization and well-child visit coding, and the challenges associated with pediatric medical coding. Answers are provided at the end for self-assessment.

Questions

1. What coding system is primarily used for documenting pediatric immunizations?

    A. ICD-10-CM

    B. CPT

    C. ICD-10-PCS

    D. HCPCS Level II

2. During a well-child visit, if a new illness is diagnosed and requires significant additional work, how should it be coded?

    A. Ignore the new diagnosis

    B. Use a preventive medicine service code only

    C. Bill separately using an appropriate E/M code

    D. Use a modifier with the well-child visit code

3. Which of the following is crucial for coding pediatric surgeries accurately?

    A. The surgeon's preference

    B. The time of day the surgery occurred

    C. Detailed surgical reports and documentation

D. The patient's favorite color

4. For inpatient pediatric procedures, which coding system is used?

A. CPT

B. ICD-10-PCS

C. HCPCS Level II

D. ICD-10-CM

5. What is a key challenge in coding for common pediatric conditions?

A. Too many codes for each condition

B. Lack of specific codes for pediatric conditions

C. Updates to vaccine codes and administration

D. Documentation specificity and completeness

6. In pediatric coding, age-specific coding considerations are important for:

A. Only determining the patient's birthday

B. Reflecting the unique healthcare needs at different stages of childhood

C. Calculating the cost of care

D. Determining the length of hospital stay

7. Immunization administration codes in pediatrics often require documentation of:

   A. Counseling provided to patients or caregivers

   B. The child's academic performance

   C. Parental employment status

   D. The weather conditions on the day of administration

8. How are preventive services, such as well-child visits, typically coded?

   A. Using ICD-10-CM codes for each preventive service

   B. With a single CPT code covering all aspects of the visit

   C. By using a separate E/M code for each service performed

   D. Preventive services are not coded

9. Coding for pediatric chronic conditions alongside acute illnesses requires:

   A. Ignoring the chronic conditions

   B. Special attention to document both conditions accurately

   C. Using only the code for the acute illness

   D. Billing for the chronic condition only

10. A significant part of pediatric coding involves:

A. Coding only for surgical procedures

B. Documentation and coding of growth and developmental milestones

C. Ignoring age-specific considerations

D. Using adult coding guidelines for all pediatric cases

Answers

1. B. CPT

2. C. Bill separately using an appropriate E/M code

3. C. Detailed surgical reports and documentation

4. B. ICD-10-PCS

5. D. Documentation specificity and completeness

6. B. Reflecting the unique healthcare needs at different stages of childhood

7. A. Counseling provided to patients or caregivers

8. B. With a single CPT code covering all aspects of the visit

9. B. Special attention to document both conditions accurately

10. B. Documentation and coding of growth and developmental milestones

These questions and answers aim to reinforce key concepts in pediatric medical coding, highlighting the importance of accurate documentation, understanding of pediatric-specific coding guidelines, and the unique challenges presented in coding for pediatric healthcare services.

Chapter 16: Specialty Coding VI: Cardiology

16.1. Cardiology Coding Fundamentals

Cardiology coding encompasses the documentation and coding of diagnostic and therapeutic procedures related to the cardiovascular system. This specialty requires an in-depth understanding of the anatomy and physiology of the heart and vascular system, as well as the specific coding guidelines for cardiology services. Accurate cardiology coding is crucial for ensuring proper reimbursement, facilitating patient care management, and contributing to cardiovascular research and quality improvement.

Key Components of Cardiology Coding

1. CPT Codes for Cardiac Procedures:

- Current Procedural Terminology (CPT) codes are used to document a wide range of cardiology procedures, including cardiac catheterizations, electrophysiological studies, pacemaker implantations, and stent placements.

2. ICD-10-CM Codes for Diagnoses:

- The International Classification of Diseases, Tenth Revision, Clinical Modification (ICD-10-CM) codes are utilized to document cardiovascular diseases and conditions, such as coronary artery disease, arrhythmias, and hypertension.

3. HCPCS Level II Codes:

- Healthcare Common Procedure Coding System (HCPCS) Level II codes may be used for products, supplies, and certain procedures not covered by CPT codes, including some medications and durable medical equipment related to cardiology care.

4. Use of Modifiers:

- Modifiers are often necessary in cardiology coding to indicate specific details about the services provided, such as bilateral procedures, multiple procedures during the same session, or services performed by more than one physician.

Challenges in Cardiology Coding

1. Complex Procedures:

- Cardiology procedures can be highly complex and involve the use of advanced technologies, requiring coders to have a detailed understanding of procedural nuances to code accurately.

2. Documentation Quality:

- Comprehensive and specific documentation is essential for supporting the codes selected, especially for high-risk and high-cost procedures. Inadequate documentation can lead to coding errors and reimbursement issues.

3. Coding Updates and Guidelines:

- Cardiology coding guidelines and the codes themselves are subject to frequent updates, necessitating continuous education and adaptation by coders.

4. Multidisciplinary Services:

- Patients receiving cardiology care often undergo procedures and treatments involving multiple specialties. Coordinating and accurately coding these multidisciplinary services can be challenging.

Strategies for Effective Cardiology Coding

1. Continuous Education and Training:

- Coders should engage in ongoing education to stay current with the latest cardiology coding practices, guidelines, and updates, particularly those related to new procedures and technologies.

2. Thorough Documentation Review:

- Carefully reviewing all documentation, including procedure reports and physician notes, is crucial for ensuring accurate and comprehensive coding of cardiology services.

3. Utilization of Coding Resources:

- Access to up-to-date coding manuals, online resources, and professional forums specializing in cardiology can aid in resolving complex coding scenarios.

4. Collaboration with Healthcare Providers:

- Effective communication with cardiologists and other healthcare providers is essential for clarifying procedural details and ensuring that documentation accurately reflects the services provided.

Conclusion

Cardiology coding is a specialized and complex area of medical coding that plays a critical role in the healthcare billing process. By mastering the fundamentals of cardiology coding, staying informed about coding updates, and employing effective coding strategies, coders can accurately document cardiovascular services, supporting the financial health of healthcare organizations and contributing to the quality of patient care.

16.2. Coding for Cardiac Procedures and Surgeries

Coding for cardiac procedures and surgeries involves the accurate representation of invasive and non-invasive treatments for heart-related conditions. This area requires a thorough understanding of the cardiovascular system, procedural techniques, and the specific coding guidelines applicable to cardiology.

Key Components in Coding Cardiac Procedures and Surgeries

1. CPT Codes for Common Cardiac Procedures:

- **Catheterization and Angiography:** Codes reflect whether the procedure is diagnostic or therapeutic, the vessels examined, and any interventions performed.

- **Pacemaker and Defibrillator Procedures:** Including implantations, replacements, and removals, each with specific codes based on the device type and approach.

- **Electrophysiological (EP) Studies and Ablation:** Coded based on the complexity of the study and the ablation technique used.

- **Coronary Artery Bypass Graft (CABG) and Valve Surgery:** Each procedure has distinct codes, reflecting the number of vessels bypassed or the type of valve surgery performed.

2. ICD-10-PCS for Inpatient Procedures:

- Used in the inpatient setting, ICD-10-PCS provides a highly detailed coding system for documenting cardiac surgeries, offering codes that specify the exact nature and techniques of the procedures.

3. ICD-10-CM Codes for Diagnoses:

- Accurate diagnosis coding using ICD-10-CM is essential for establishing the medical necessity of cardiac procedures and surgeries.

4. Use of Modifiers:

- Modifiers may be necessary to indicate specific circumstances of the procedures, such as bilateral procedures, staged or related procedures performed during the same operative session, or procedures performed by more than one physician.

Challenges in Coding for Cardiac Procedures and Surgeries

1. Procedure Complexity:

- The complexity and variety of cardiac procedures require coders to have an in-depth understanding of each procedure's nuances to select the appropriate codes accurately.

2. Rapid Technological Advances:

- Cardiology is a field characterized by rapid innovation and the introduction of new procedures and devices, necessitating continuous learning and adaptation by coders.

3. Documentation Specificity:

- Detailed procedural documentation is crucial but can be challenging to obtain. Coders often need to collaborate closely with healthcare providers to ensure that all necessary details are accurately documented.

4. Multidisciplinary Nature:

- Cardiac care often involves multiple specialties and procedures. Coordinating and accurately coding these services to reflect the comprehensive care provided can be complex.

Strategies for Effective Coding of Cardiac Procedures and Surgeries

1. Specialized Training and Education:

- Coders specializing in cardiology should pursue ongoing education focused on cardiac procedures, coding updates, and the impact of new technologies on coding practices.

2. Utilization of Specialized Coding Resources:

- Access to cardiology-specific coding manuals, online databases, and forums can help coders resolve complex coding issues and stay updated on coding changes.

3. Collaboration with Cardiology Teams:

- Establishing strong communication channels with cardiologists and surgical teams ensures that coders have access to comprehensive and accurate documentation for coding.

4. Regular Coding Audits:

- Conducting periodic audits of cardiac procedure coding can help identify coding errors, areas for improvement, and opportunities for coder education.

Conclusion

Accurate coding for cardiac procedures and surgeries is essential for proper reimbursement, patient care management, and compliance with healthcare regulations. By employing targeted strategies to address the unique challenges of cardiology coding, coders can ensure that cardiovascular services are accurately documented and coded, supporting the financial and clinical goals of healthcare organizations.

16.3. Diagnostic Testing in Cardiology Coding

Diagnostic testing plays a crucial role in cardiology, aiding in the detection, assessment, and management of heart-related conditions. Coding for these tests requires specific knowledge of the procedures involved and the appropriate use of coding systems to accurately document the services provided.

Key Components of Diagnostic Testing in Cardiology Coding

1. CPT Codes for Diagnostic Procedures:

- **Echocardiograms:** Codes differentiate between transthoracic, transesophageal, and stress echocardiography, reflecting the complexity and technique used.

- **Electrocardiograms (EKGs):** Coded based on the number of leads recorded and whether an interpretation and report are included.

- **Stress Tests:** Codes vary depending on whether the test is exercise-induced or pharmacologically induced, and if imaging is used.

- **Holter Monitoring and Event Recorders:** The duration of monitoring and the type of device used influence the coding.

- **Cardiac Catheterization:** Includes diagnostic catheterizations and angiographies, coded based on the vessels examined and procedures performed during catheterization.

2. ICD-10-CM Codes for Diagnoses:

- Diagnosis coding using ICD-10-CM supports the medical necessity of the diagnostic test, linking the patient's condition to the need for the procedure.

3. Modifiers:

- Modifiers may be required to indicate specific circumstances of the testing, such as repeat or multiple tests, tests performed bilaterally, or when tests are part of a global service.

Challenges in Coding for Diagnostic Testing in Cardiology

1. Understanding Test Variations:

- The variety of diagnostic tests and their specific applications can make coding complex, requiring detailed knowledge of cardiology procedures.

2. Keeping Up with Technology and Guidelines:

- Advances in diagnostic technologies and changes in coding guidelines necessitate continuous education to ensure coding accuracy.

3. Documentation Requirements:

- Detailed documentation is essential for justifying the test's medical necessity and ensuring the selection of accurate codes.

Inadequate documentation can lead to coding errors and claim denials.

4. Differentiating Between Screening and Diagnostic Tests:

- Coding differs between screening tests performed for preventive reasons and diagnostic tests conducted to evaluate specific symptoms or conditions, which can be a source of confusion.

Strategies for Effective Diagnostic Testing Coding in Cardiology

1. Specialized Training and Continuing Education:

- Coders should engage in ongoing training specific to cardiology diagnostic testing, focusing on procedural details and coding updates.

2. Utilize Coding Resources and Tools:

- Access to current coding manuals, online resources, and professional forums specializing in cardiology can aid in resolving coding questions and staying informed about changes.

3. Collaboration with Healthcare Providers:

- Effective communication with cardiologists and technicians ensures that coders have access to detailed procedure reports and clarifications necessary for accurate coding.

4. Regular Review and Auditing:

- Conducting regular audits of diagnostic testing coding practices can identify areas for improvement, reduce the risk of errors, and enhance compliance with coding standards.

Conclusion

Coding for diagnostic testing in cardiology is a critical component of medical coding that requires an understanding of both the technical aspects of cardiology procedures and the intricacies of coding systems. By employing targeted strategies to address the challenges associated with coding these procedures, coders can ensure accurate documentation and reimbursement for diagnostic services, ultimately supporting patient care and the financial health of healthcare organizations.

16.4. Coding Challenges in Cardiology

Cardiology, with its intricate procedures and rapidly advancing technologies, presents unique coding challenges. These challenges not only test the coders' knowledge and adaptability but also underscore the importance of precise coding to ensure accurate reimbursement and compliance with healthcare regulations.

Key Challenges in Cardiology Coding

1. Procedure Complexity and Specificity:

- Cardiology procedures can be highly complex, involving detailed techniques and technologies. Accurately capturing every aspect of these procedures requires a deep understanding of cardiology-specific coding guidelines.

2. Rapid Advancements in Technology:

- The cardiology field is at the forefront of medical innovation, introducing new procedures, devices, and treatment modalities. Keeping up with these advancements and understanding how they translate into coding practices can be daunting.

3. Multi-component Procedures:

- Many cardiology procedures involve multiple steps or components, each of which may need separate coding. Distinguishing between bundled and separately billable components requires careful attention to coding rules.

4. Documentation Requirements:

- Detailed and precise documentation is crucial for supporting the codes selected for cardiology services. Inadequate or unclear documentation can lead to coding errors, claim denials, or compliance issues.

5. Use of Modifiers:

- Modifiers play a significant role in cardiology coding, indicating nuances such as bilateral procedures, multiple procedures, or services performed by more than one provider. Incorrect use of modifiers can impact reimbursement.

6. Distinguishing Between Diagnostic and Therapeutic Procedures:

- Coding differs for diagnostic and therapeutic procedures, even when the procedures appear similar. Determining the intent and outcome of the procedure is essential for correct code assignment.

Strategies to Overcome Coding Challenges in Cardiology

1. Continuous Education and Training:

- Engaging in ongoing education, including attending workshops, webinars, and conferences focused on cardiology coding, is vital to stay current with coding guidelines and technological advancements.

2. Utilization of Specialized Coding Resources:

- Accessing cardiology-specific coding manuals, online databases, and forums can help coders resolve complex coding issues and stay informed about changes in coding practices.

3. Collaboration with Cardiology Teams:

- Establishing strong communication channels with cardiologists, surgeons, and other medical professionals ensures access to detailed procedural information, aiding accurate coding.

4. Regular Documentation Audits:

- Conducting periodic audits of cardiology coding and documentation practices helps identify areas for improvement, enhancing accuracy and compliance.

5. Leveraging Coding Software and Tools:

- Advanced coding software and tools that include up-to-date cardiology coding guidelines and edits can assist in accurate code selection and error reduction.

6. Networking with Peers:

- Participating in professional coding associations and forums allows for the exchange of knowledge and experiences with peers, offering additional insights and solutions to common challenges.

Conclusion

The dynamic and complex nature of cardiology requires coders to adopt a proactive approach to education, utilize available resources, and foster collaboration with healthcare providers. By addressing the unique coding challenges in cardiology, coders can ensure accurate documentation and coding of cardiology services, supporting optimal patient care and the financial sustainability of healthcare organizations.

16.5. Exercise: 10 MCQs with Answers at the End

Test your knowledge on Specialty Coding VI: Cardiology, covering cardiology coding fundamentals, coding for cardiac procedures and surgeries, diagnostic testing in cardiology, and the challenges associated with cardiology medical coding. Answers are provided at the end for self-assessment.

Questions

1. What coding system is primarily used for documenting cardiac catheterization procedures?

A. ICD-10-CM

B. CPT

C. ICD-10-PCS

D. HCPCS Level II

2. In cardiology coding, which modifier might be used to indicate a procedure performed bilaterally?

A. -50

B. -25

C. -59

D. -LT and -RT

3. The coding of a pacemaker insertion procedure would primarily use which of the following code sets?

A. ICD-10-CM

B. CPT

C. ICD-10-PCS

D. HCPCS Level II

4. Which of the following is a challenge in coding for cardiology procedures?

A. Lack of specific codes for cardiac procedures

B. Procedure complexity and specificity

C. Simplistic nature of cardiac surgeries

D. Abundance of clear, concise documentation

5. Diagnostic tests in cardiology, like echocardiograms, are coded using:

    A. ICD-10-PCS codes

    B. CPT codes

    C. ICD-10-CM codes

    D. HCPCS Level II codes

6. Accurate documentation in cardiology coding is crucial for:

    A. Reducing the number of procedures performed

    B. Supporting the codes selected for services provided

    C. Increasing patient wait times

    D. Simplifying healthcare policies

7. The use of ICD-10-CM codes in cardiology coding is primarily for:

    A. Documenting procedures

    B. Reporting diagnoses

    C. Indicating modifiers

    D. Specifying the location of the hospital

8. A key strategy to overcome challenges in cardiology coding is:

    A. Decreasing collaboration with healthcare providers

    B. Limiting access to coding resources and tools

C. Engaging in continuous education and training

D. Ignoring updates to coding guidelines and technologies

9. Coding for a stress test that includes imaging would require:

A. Only a single CPT code for stress testing

B. Separate CPT codes for the stress test and imaging component

C. An ICD-10-CM code for stress

D. A HCPCS Level II code for the treadmill

10. In cardiology coding, distinguishing between diagnostic and therapeutic procedures is important because:

A. It impacts the patient's diagnosis

B. It affects the choice of treatment

C. It influences code selection and reimbursement

D. It determines the length of the hospital stay

Answers

1. B. CPT

2. A. -50

3. B. CPT

4. B. Procedure complexity and specificity

5. B. CPT codes

6. B. Supporting the codes selected for services provided

7. B. Reporting diagnoses

8. C. Engaging in continuous education and training

9. B. Separate CPT codes for the stress test and imaging component

10. C. It influences code selection and reimbursement

These questions and answers aim to reinforce key concepts in cardiology coding, highlighting the importance of accurate coding practices, the challenges encountered, and the strategies employed to ensure compliance and appropriate reimbursement for cardiology services.

Chapter 17: Specialty Coding VII: Orthopedics

17.1. Orthopedic Coding Overview

Orthopedic coding involves the documentation and coding of medical services related to the diagnosis, treatment, and management of disorders, injuries, and conditions affecting the musculoskeletal system. This specialty requires a thorough understanding of anatomy, surgical procedures, and the specific coding guidelines applicable to orthopedics. Accurate orthopedic coding is crucial for ensuring proper reimbursement, facilitating patient care management, and contributing to healthcare data collection and analysis.

Key Aspects of Orthopedic Coding

1. CPT Codes for Orthopedic Procedures:

- Orthopedic procedures are primarily coded using Current Procedural Terminology (CPT) codes. These include codes for surgeries related to fractures, joint replacements, arthroscopies, and repairs of ligament and tendon injuries.

2. ICD-10-CM Codes for Diagnoses:

- The International Classification of Diseases, Tenth Revision, Clinical Modification (ICD-10-CM) is used to document orthopedic diagnoses, including fractures, dislocations, osteoarthritis, and other musculoskeletal conditions.

3. HCPCS Level II Codes:

- HCPCS Level II codes may be used for orthopedic devices, durable medical equipment, and certain injectable drugs not covered by CPT codes.

4. Use of Modifiers:

- Modifiers are critical in orthopedic coding to indicate specifics such as laterality, staged or related procedures, and services provided by more than one physician.

Challenges in Orthopedic Coding

1. Procedure Complexity:

- Orthopedic surgeries can be highly complex, often involving multiple steps or components that need accurate coding to reflect the full scope of the procedure.

2. Detailed Documentation:

- Comprehensive and specific documentation is essential for supporting the codes selected, especially for procedures with multiple surgical sites or techniques.

3. Keeping Up with Coding Updates:

- Orthopedic coding guidelines and the codes themselves are subject to frequent updates, necessitating continuous education and adaptation by coders.

4. Laterality and Specificity:

- Many orthopedic conditions and injuries are specific to certain limbs or sides of the body, requiring careful attention to laterality and specificity in coding.

Strategies for Effective Orthopedic Coding

1. Continuous Education and Training:

- Coders specializing in orthopedics should engage in ongoing education to stay current with the latest coding practices, guidelines, and updates relevant to orthopedic procedures.

2. Thorough Documentation Review:

- Carefully reviewing all documentation, including operative reports and physician notes, is crucial for ensuring accurate and comprehensive coding of orthopedic services.

3. Utilization of Coding Resources:

- Access to up-to-date coding manuals, online resources, and professional forums specializing in orthopedics can aid in resolving complex coding scenarios.

4. Collaboration with Healthcare Providers:

- Establishing effective communication with orthopedic surgeons and other healthcare providers is essential for clarifying procedural details and ensuring that documentation accurately reflects the services provided.

Conclusion

Orthopedic coding is a specialized and complex area of medical coding that plays a critical role in the healthcare billing process. By mastering the fundamentals of orthopedic coding, staying informed about coding updates, and employing effective coding strategies, coders can accurately document orthopedic services, supporting the financial health of healthcare organizations and the quality of patient care.

17.2. Coding for Orthopedic Surgeries and Procedures

Orthopedic surgeries and procedures encompass a wide range of treatments for disorders and injuries affecting the musculoskeletal system. Accurate coding of these procedures is essential for appropriate reimbursement, healthcare management, and quality reporting.

Key Components in Coding Orthopedic Surgeries and Procedures

1. Surgical Procedure Coding with CPT:

- **Fracture Care:** CPT codes for fracture care often include the treatment (e.g., closed, open, or percutaneous fixation) and the specific bone or location of the fracture. Global fracture care codes cover all related care from the day of surgery through the recovery period.

- **Joint Procedures:** This includes arthroscopies, reconstructions, replacements, and repairs, with specific codes based on the joint involved and the type of procedure performed.

- **Spinal Surgeries:** Coding for spinal procedures requires detailed information about the anatomical location, approach (anterior, posterior, or lateral), and any instrumentation or fusion materials used.

2. Use of ICD-10-PCS for Inpatient Procedures:

- In the inpatient setting, ICD-10-PCS codes provide a highly detailed system for documenting orthopedic surgeries, offering specificity regarding the approach, device, and body part.

3. Diagnosis Coding with ICD-10-CM:

- Accurate diagnosis coding using ICD-10-CM is crucial for establishing the medical necessity of orthopedic procedures. This includes coding for acute injuries, chronic conditions, and post-surgical complications.

4. Modifiers to Indicate Specific Circumstances:

- Modifiers are used to convey additional information about the procedure, such as laterality, multiple procedures during the same session, or staged procedures.

Challenges in Coding Orthopedic Surgeries and Procedures

1. Procedure Complexity and Specificity:

- The detailed nature of orthopedic surgeries requires coders to understand the specifics of each procedure, including the technique used and any devices or grafts implanted.

2. Documentation Requirements:

- Comprehensive operative reports and clinical documentation are essential for accurate coding but can be challenging to decipher, especially with complex surgeries.

3. Keeping Up with Advances:

- Orthopedics is a rapidly evolving field with continual advancements in surgical techniques and devices, necessitating ongoing education for coders to remain current.

4. Global Billing Issues:

- Understanding what is included in global surgery packages versus what can be billed separately is a common challenge in orthopedic coding.

Strategies for Effective Coding of Orthopedic Surgeries and Procedures

1. Continuous Education and Specialization:

- Coders should pursue specialized training in orthopedic coding and stay updated on the latest procedural codes and guidelines.

2. Detailed Documentation Review:

- Thoroughly review surgical reports and patient records to ensure that all aspects of the procedure are accurately documented and coded.

3. Use of Orthopedic Coding Resources:

- Leverage specialized orthopedic coding manuals, online databases, and professional networks to clarify coding queries and stay informed about coding updates.

4. Collaboration with Orthopedic Surgeons and Staff:

- Foster open communication with the surgical team to clarify procedural details and ensure complete understanding of the surgeries performed.

Conclusion

Coding for orthopedic surgeries and procedures requires a detailed understanding of musculoskeletal anatomy, surgical techniques, and coding guidelines. By addressing the challenges through education, thorough documentation review, and collaboration with healthcare providers, coders can achieve accurate and efficient coding in orthopedics, enhancing reimbursement and supporting high-quality patient care.

17.3. Musculoskeletal System Coding Challenges

Coding for the musculoskeletal system in orthopedics involves documenting treatments for a wide array of conditions affecting bones, joints, and soft tissues. This specialty area presents several challenges that require precision and a deep understanding of both the anatomy and the specific coding guidelines.

Key Challenges in Musculoskeletal System Coding

1. Anatomical Specificity:

- The musculoskeletal system encompasses a vast array of structures, each with its coding nuances. Coders must accurately capture the specific anatomy involved, including laterality and the exact bone, joint, or muscle.

2. Procedure Complexity:

- Orthopedic procedures range from simple fracture repairs to complex joint reconstructions and spine surgeries. Each procedure type has its coding requirements, which can be challenging to navigate.

3. Global Periods and Bundled Services:

- Understanding what is included in the global surgical package versus what can be billed separately is crucial. Procedures performed within the global period of another service may not be separately billable unless they meet specific criteria.

4. Use of Modifiers:

- Proper application of modifiers is critical in orthopedic coding to indicate services that are distinct or outside the global surgical package. Misuse of modifiers can lead to claim denials or incorrect reimbursement.

5. Documentation and Support for Medical Necessity:

- Detailed operative reports and medical records are essential to support the use of specific codes. Coders often face challenges with incomplete or nonspecific documentation, making it difficult to justify the coding choices.

6. Advances in Surgical Techniques and Technologies:

- Orthopedics is a rapidly evolving field, with new procedures and technologies constantly emerging. Keeping up-to-date with these advances and understanding how they affect coding practices is a significant challenge.

Strategies to Overcome Coding Challenges

1. Specialized Training:

- Invest in ongoing education and training focused on orthopedic coding, including anatomy, procedural details, and coding updates, to enhance accuracy and efficiency.

2. Thorough Documentation Review:

- Carefully review all available documentation to ensure a comprehensive understanding of the services provided. Query physicians or surgeons for clarification when necessary.

3. Utilize Authoritative Resources:

- Access up-to-date coding manuals, online resources, and professional associations to stay informed about current coding guidelines and best practices in orthopedics.

4. Regular Auditing and Quality Checks:

- Implement regular coding audits to identify and address common errors or inconsistencies. Use audit findings to inform targeted education and process improvements.

5. Collaboration with Healthcare Providers:

- Foster collaborative relationships with orthopedic surgeons and other healthcare providers to ensure accurate documentation and to clarify ambiguous or complex cases.

Conclusion

Coding for the musculoskeletal system presents unique challenges that demand a specialized skill set and an in-depth knowledge of orthopedic procedures and coding guidelines. By adopting targeted strategies to address these challenges, coders can ensure accurate and compliant coding, supporting optimal reimbursement and contributing to the delivery of high-quality orthopedic care.

17.4. Coding for Orthopedic Trauma and Fractures

Coding for orthopedic trauma and fractures is a critical aspect of medical billing in the field of orthopedics. These cases often involve emergency care, surgical treatment, and long-term management, requiring coders to navigate a complex set of coding guidelines to accurately document these services.

Key Components in Coding Orthopedic Trauma and Fractures

1. CPT Codes for Fracture Treatment:

- **Closed vs. Open Treatment:** Codes differ based on whether the fracture treatment was closed (without an incision) or open (requiring surgical exposure of the fracture).

- **Percutaneous Skeletal Fixation:** Used when fractures are treated with hardware insertion without fully opening the site.

- **External Fixation:** Involves the stabilization of fractures with external devices, requiring specific coding based on the complexity and method of fixation.

2. ICD-10-CM Codes for Fracture Diagnoses:

- Fracture coding in ICD-10-CM includes codes that specify the fracture's location, type, and whether it is initial or subsequent care. It also considers the healing status of the fracture.

3. Global Surgical Package:

- Many fracture treatments are considered part of a global surgical package, which includes all the necessary services normally furnished by a surgeon before, during, and after a procedure.

4. Use of Modifiers:

- Modifiers are essential in orthopedic trauma and fracture coding to indicate specific circumstances like multiple fractures, bilateral injuries, or services provided outside the global period.

Challenges in Coding for Orthopedic Trauma and Fractures

1. Detail and Specificity Requirements:

- Accurate fracture coding requires detailed information about the fracture's location, type, and the treatment provided, which can be challenging to decipher from medical records.

2. Managing Global Periods:

- Understanding and managing the global surgical package for fracture care, including what services are included or billable separately, can be complex.

3. Staying Updated with Coding Changes:

- Orthopedic coding guidelines, particularly for trauma and fractures, are subject to frequent updates. Coders must stay informed to ensure compliance and accurate billing.

4. Documentation Gaps:

- Incomplete or ambiguous documentation from healthcare providers can pose significant challenges, potentially leading to coding inaccuracies and claim denials.

Strategies for Effective Coding of Orthopedic Trauma and Fractures

1. Continuous Education:

- Engage in ongoing education and training specific to orthopedic coding to stay current with the latest guidelines and coding practices.

2. Detailed Documentation Review:

- Thoroughly review medical records for precise details about the fracture and treatment, and query providers for missing information or clarification as needed.

3. Utilize Authoritative Coding Resources:

- Leverage up-to-date coding manuals, online databases, and orthopedic coding forums to access expert advice and clarify complex coding scenarios.

4. Monitor and Apply Coding Updates:

- Regularly review coding updates from authoritative sources such as the AMA and CMS to ensure coding practices are aligned with current standards.

5. Collaboration with Healthcare Providers:

- Foster collaborative relationships with orthopedic surgeons and medical staff to improve documentation quality and ensure accurate representation of the care provided.

Conclusion

Coding for orthopedic trauma and fractures demands a high level of expertise and attention to detail, given the complexity of cases and the specificity required in documentation. By implementing targeted strategies to address coding challenges, coders can enhance accuracy, compliance, and reimbursement for orthopedic services, ultimately supporting effective patient care management.

17.5. Exercise: 10 MCQs with Answers at the End

Test your knowledge on Specialty Coding VII: Orthopedics, focusing on orthopedic coding overview, coding for orthopedic surgeries and procedures, musculoskeletal system coding challenges, coding for orthopedic trauma and fractures, and the challenges associated with orthopedic medical coding. Answers are provided at the end for self-assessment.

Questions

1. What coding system is primarily used for documenting orthopedic surgeries?

   A. ICD-10-CM

   B. CPT

   C. ICD-10-PCS

   D. HCPCS Level II

2. In orthopedic coding, a modifier might be used to indicate:

   A. The patient's age

   B. A procedure performed bilaterally

   C. The time of day the procedure was performed

   D. The patient's insurance type

3. Which code set is used for inpatient orthopedic procedure documentation?

A. CPT

B. ICD-10-CM

C. ICD-10-PCS

D. HCPCS Level II

4. A key challenge in orthopedic coding is:

A. The oversimplification of procedures

B. The frequent under-documentation of services

C. Procedure complexity and specificity

D. A lack of available modifiers

5. The global surgical package for fracture care typically includes:

A. Only the initial consultation

B. The surgical procedure only, without follow-up care

C. All related care from the day of surgery through the recovery period

D. Post-operative care only

6. Documentation for orthopedic trauma coding must specifically include:

A. The color of the cast used

B. Location, type, and treatment of the fracture

C. The patient's dietary preferences

D. The number of visitors the patient had

7. Coding updates in orthopedics are challenging because:

A. They rarely occur

B. They are too simple to understand

C. They require re-learning anatomy

D. They necessitate continuous education to stay current

8. Effective strategies for orthopedic coding do NOT include:

A. Ignoring updates to coding guidelines

B. Engaging in continuous education

C. Utilizing authoritative coding resources

D. Collaboration with healthcare providers

9. ICD-10-CM codes in orthopedic coding are primarily used for:

A. Reporting diagnoses

B. Documenting surgical procedures

C. Indicating the use of equipment

D. Specifying the hospital department

10. Modifiers in orthopedic coding help to indicate:

A. The severity of the patient's pain

B. Specific circumstances surrounding a procedure

C. The length of the hospital stay

D. The patient's mood during the procedure

Answers

1. B. CPT

2. B. A procedure performed bilaterally

3. C. ICD-10-PCS

4. C. Procedure complexity and specificity

5. C. All related care from the day of surgery through the recovery period

6. B. Location, type, and treatment of the fracture

7. D. They necessitate continuous education to stay current

8. A. Ignoring updates to coding guidelines

9. A. Reporting diagnoses

10. B. Specific circumstances surrounding a procedure

Chapter 18: Specialty Coding VIII: Oncology

18.1. Oncology Coding Basics

Oncology coding encompasses the documentation and coding of medical services related to the diagnosis, treatment, and management of cancer. This specialized area of medical coding requires a comprehensive understanding of oncology procedures, treatments (including chemotherapy, radiation therapy, and surgical interventions), and the unique coding guidelines applicable to cancer care.

Key Aspects of Oncology Coding

1. ICD-10-CM Codes for Cancer Diagnoses:

- Accurate diagnosis coding is crucial in oncology, using the International Classification of Diseases, Tenth Revision, Clinical Modification (ICD-10-CM). Codes should reflect the type, location, and behavior of the neoplasm, as well as any associated conditions or complications.

2. CPT and HCPCS Codes for Oncology Treatments:

- **Chemotherapy and Immunotherapy:** Coding for these treatments involves specific CPT and HCPCS codes that indicate the drugs administered, the method of administration, and any supportive care provided.

- **Radiation Therapy:** Includes codes for the planning, delivery, and management of radiation treatment.

- **Surgical Procedures:** Coded using CPT codes that correspond to the surgical intervention performed to treat or manage cancer.

3. Modifiers in Oncology Coding:

- Modifiers are used to provide additional information about the services rendered, such as whether a procedure was performed bilaterally or if multiple sessions of a therapy were conducted.

Challenges in Oncology Coding

1. Complexity of Cancer Treatment:

- Oncology coding is challenged by the complex nature of cancer treatment protocols, which often involve a combination of surgery, chemotherapy, and radiation therapy.

2. Specificity of Diagnosis Codes:

- The specificity required in coding cancer diagnoses can be challenging, necessitating detailed documentation about the type, origin, and behavior of the neoplasm.

3. Coding for Chemotherapy Regimens:

- Chemotherapy involves numerous drugs and regimens, each with specific coding requirements. Keeping track of the codes for new drugs and combination therapies can be difficult.

4. Documentation and Medical Necessity:

- Comprehensive documentation that supports the medical necessity of each treatment is essential for accurate coding and reimbursement.

Strategies for Effective Oncology Coding

1. Continuous Education and Training:

- Oncology coders should pursue ongoing education to stay current with the latest coding guidelines, treatment protocols, and advancements in cancer care.

2. Detailed Documentation Review:

- Thoroughly review medical records to ensure accurate and comprehensive documentation of the diagnosis, treatment plan, and services provided.

3. Utilization of Coding Resources:

- Leverage specialized oncology coding manuals, online databases, and forums to access expert advice and clarify complex coding scenarios.

4. Collaboration with Healthcare Providers:

- Establish strong communication with oncologists and cancer care teams to clarify treatment details and ensure the accuracy of coding.

Conclusion

Oncology coding is a critical component of the healthcare billing process, requiring a specialized skill set to navigate the complexities of cancer diagnosis and treatment coding. By implementing effective coding strategies and staying informed about the latest developments in oncology care, coders can ensure accurate documentation and reimbursement, ultimately supporting the delivery of high-quality cancer care.

18.2. Coding for Cancer Treatments and Procedures

Coding for cancer treatments and procedures is a vital part of oncology coding, encompassing a broad range of services from diagnostic testing to complex treatments such as chemotherapy, radiation therapy, and surgical interventions. Accurate coding is essential for reimbursement and for documenting the care provided to patients with cancer.

Key Aspects of Coding for Cancer Treatments and Procedures

1. Chemotherapy and Immunotherapy Coding:

- **CPT and HCPCS Codes:** Specific codes are used for the administration of chemotherapy and immunotherapy, including intravenous infusions, injections, and oral chemotherapy. HCPCS codes are particularly important for identifying the specific drugs administered.

- **Modifiers:** Modifiers may be necessary to indicate specific details about the chemotherapy administration, such as concurrent infusion or the use of a pump for continuous infusion.

2. Radiation Therapy Coding:

- **Treatment Planning:** Codes cover the initial and ongoing treatment planning, including simulations and dosimetry calculations.

- **Delivery Techniques:** Coding varies based on the delivery method, such as external beam radiation, intensity-modulated radiation therapy (IMRT), or brachytherapy. Each technique has specific codes.

- **Management:** Codes are also used for the management and follow-up during the course of radiation treatment.

3. Surgical Procedures in Oncology:

- **CPT Codes:** Surgical interventions for cancer, including biopsies, tumor removals, and reconstructive surgeries, are coded using CPT codes. The codes chosen depend on the surgical site, the extent of the procedure, and any reconstructive efforts.

- **Modifiers:** Surgical coding may require modifiers to indicate procedures performed on multiple sites or to address surgeries that are part of a larger treatment plan.

Challenges in Coding for Cancer Treatments and Procedures

1. Multidisciplinary Treatment Plans:

- Patients with cancer often receive care from multiple specialists, complicating the coding process with overlapping and concurrent treatments.

2. Keeping Up with Advances in Treatment:

- The rapid development of new cancer treatments and technologies requires coders to continuously update their knowledge to accurately code these interventions.

3. Documentation of Treatment Protocols:

- Detailed documentation is necessary to support the use of specific treatment codes, particularly for chemotherapy regimens and radiation therapy plans.

4. Specificity and Accuracy:

- Coding for cancer treatments requires a high level of specificity to accurately reflect the services provided, necessitating precise documentation and coding expertise.

Strategies for Effective Coding of Cancer Treatments and Procedures

1. Continuous Education:

- Engage in ongoing education focused on oncology coding, including seminars, workshops, and certification courses, to stay current with treatment advances and coding guidelines.

2. Collaboration with Oncology Teams:

- Work closely with oncologists, pharmacists, and radiation therapists to ensure comprehensive understanding and documentation of cancer treatments.

3. Utilize Specialized Resources:

- Access oncology-specific coding manuals, databases, and professional forums to find guidance on complex coding scenarios and updates to treatment codes.

4. Detailed Review of Medical Records:

- Conduct thorough reviews of patient records, treatment plans, and provider notes to ensure accurate coding of the treatments administered.

Conclusion

Coding for cancer treatments and procedures requires an in-depth understanding of oncology, meticulous attention to detail, and a commitment to continuous learning. By employing effective strategies and maintaining open communication with healthcare providers, coders can accurately document cancer care, supporting optimal patient outcomes and ensuring appropriate reimbursement.

18.3. Hematology and Chemotherapy Coding

Hematology and chemotherapy coding involves documenting treatments for blood disorders and cancer using pharmaceuticals. This specialized coding area requires detailed knowledge of the drugs used, administration methods, and the coding guidelines that apply to these treatments. Accurate coding ensures appropriate reimbursement and reflects the care's complexity and intensity provided to patients.

Key Components of Hematology and Chemotherapy Coding

1. HCPCS Level II Codes for Drugs:

- Each chemotherapy and hematology medication has a specific HCPCS Level II code that identifies the drug administered. These codes are crucial for billing and reimbursement purposes, as they denote the specific pharmaceuticals used in treatment.

2. CPT Codes for Administration:

- The administration of chemotherapy and hematology treatments involves specific CPT codes that describe how the treatment was delivered (e.g., intravenous infusion, subcutaneous injection). These codes are selected based on the administration's complexity, duration, and setting.

3. ICD-10-CM Codes for Diagnoses:

- Accurate diagnostic coding using ICD-10-CM is essential to establish medical necessity for chemotherapy and hematology treatments. Codes should reflect the patient's primary diagnosis, any secondary conditions, and the reason for the treatment.

4. Modifiers to Indicate Specific Circumstances:

- Modifiers are used in hematology and chemotherapy coding to provide additional details about the treatment, such as whether it's an initial or subsequent encounter, or if multiple drugs are administered during the same session.

Challenges in Hematology and Chemotherapy Coding

1. Complexity of Regimens:

- Chemotherapy and hematology treatments often involve complex regimens with multiple drugs, dosages, and administration routes, making coding challenging.

2. Documentation Requirements:

- Detailed documentation is necessary to justify the use of specific drugs and administration codes. Incomplete or unclear documentation can lead to coding errors and reimbursement issues.

3. Keeping Up with Drug Codes:

- New drugs are frequently introduced, and existing drugs may have coding changes. Staying updated on these changes is crucial for accurate coding.

4. Coding for Combination Therapies:

- Patients may receive combination therapies that require careful coding to accurately capture all aspects of the treatment provided.

**Strategies for Effective Hematology and Chemotherapy Coding

1. Continuous Education and Training:

- Coders should engage in ongoing education focused on oncology and hematology coding, including updates to drug codes and administration methods.

2. Detailed Review of Documentation:

- Thoroughly review treatment plans, physician orders, and administration records to ensure all aspects of the treatment are accurately documented and coded.

3. Use of Authoritative Resources:

- Utilize up-to-date coding manuals, online databases, and professional forums to stay informed about the latest coding guidelines and drug codes.

4. Collaboration with Healthcare Providers:

- Work closely with oncologists, hematologists, and pharmacy staff to clarify treatment details and ensure accurate representation of the care provided.

Conclusion

Hematology and chemotherapy coding is a critical component of oncology coding, requiring specialized knowledge and attention to detail. By implementing effective coding practices and staying informed about the latest treatment advances and coding updates, coders can accurately document these complex treatments, supporting optimal patient care and appropriate reimbursement.

18.4. Challenges in Oncology Coding

Oncology coding, given its complexity and the critical nature of cancer care, presents several unique challenges. Accurate coding is essential not only for reimbursement purposes but also for patient care management, reporting, and compliance with healthcare regulations.

Key Challenges in Oncology Coding

1. Complexity of Cancer Treatment Regimens:

- Cancer treatment often involves a multidisciplinary approach, including surgery, chemotherapy, radiation therapy, and targeted therapies. Each treatment type requires specific coding, and treatments may change over time as the patient's condition evolves.

2. Specificity of Diagnosis Codes:

- ICD-10-CM codes for oncology are highly specific, requiring detailed information about the type, location, and behavior of the neoplasm. Coders must accurately capture this information to ensure proper coding and reimbursement.

3. Coding for Chemotherapy and Other Drug Therapies:

- The coding of chemotherapy and other drug therapies involves not only the selection of the appropriate HCPCS codes for the drugs administered but also the correct CPT codes for the administration of these drugs. New drugs frequently enter the market, and existing drugs may have changes in indications or dosages, adding to the complexity.

4. Documentation Requirements:

- Comprehensive documentation is essential to support the coding of oncology services. This includes detailed information on the diagnosis, treatment plan, administration of therapies, and any adverse reactions or complications.

5. Modifier Use:

- Modifiers play a crucial role in oncology coding to indicate specific circumstances of the care provided. Incorrect use of modifiers can lead to claim denials or incorrect reimbursement.

6. Staying Updated with Coding Guidelines and Regulations:

- Oncology coding guidelines and payer policies are subject to frequent changes. Coders must stay informed about these updates to ensure compliance and accurate billing.

Strategies to Overcome Challenges in Oncology Coding

1. Continuous Education and Training:

- Invest in ongoing education for coders, focusing on oncology-specific coding practices, updates to coding guidelines, and new treatment modalities.

2. Thorough Documentation Review:

- Conduct detailed reviews of medical records to ensure all necessary information is captured for accurate coding. This may involve querying physicians for additional details or clarification.

3. Utilization of Specialized Resources:

- Access oncology-specific coding manuals, databases, and professional societies that offer resources and forums for coders to discuss complex cases and stay updated on industry changes.

4. Collaboration with Healthcare Providers:

- Establish strong communication channels with oncologists, pharmacists, and other members of the cancer care team to ensure coding accuracy and to clarify treatment details.

5. Regular Auditing and Quality Checks:

- Implement regular coding audits to identify areas for improvement, reduce the risk of errors, and enhance compliance with coding standards and payer policies.

Conclusion

Oncology coding is fraught with challenges that demand a high level of expertise, meticulous attention to detail, and a proactive approach to education and training. By employing targeted strategies to address these challenges, coders can ensure accurate and compliant coding, supporting the financial health of healthcare organizations and the effective management of patient care in the field of oncology.

18.5. Exercise: 10 MCQs with Answers at the End

Test your understanding of Specialty Coding VIII: Oncology, covering oncology coding basics, coding for cancer treatments and procedures, hematology and chemotherapy coding, and the challenges associated with oncology medical coding. Answers are provided at the end for self-assessment.

Questions

1. What coding system is primarily used for documenting the administration of chemotherapy?

    A. ICD-10-CM

    B. CPT

    C. ICD-10-PCS

    D. HCPCS Level II

2. The specificity of ICD-10-CM codes for oncology requires detailed information about:

   A. The cost of treatment

   B. The type, location, and behavior of the neoplasm

   C. The patient's insurance provider

   D. The hospital's location

3. HCPCS Level II codes are essential in oncology coding for:

   A. Surgical procedures

   B. Radiation therapy sessions

   C. Identifying specific chemotherapy drugs

   D. Documentation of patient counseling

4. A key challenge in oncology coding is:

   A. The simplicity of treatment regimens

   B. Staying updated with coding guidelines and regulations

   C. A lack of available codes for cancer treatments

   D. Over-documentation by healthcare providers

5. In oncology, modifiers are used to indicate:

   A. The color of medication

B. Specific circumstances of the care provided

C. The number of days in the treatment cycle

D. The dietary preferences of the patient

6. Continuous education and training for coders in oncology are crucial for:

A. Learning basic coding skills

B. Staying informed about new treatment modalities and coding updates

C. Reducing the workload

D. Avoiding communication with healthcare providers

7. Coding for radiation therapy involves:

A. Only the use of ICD-10-CM codes

B. CPT codes for treatment planning, delivery, and management

C. HCPCS Level II codes for the machines used

D. Modifiers for the type of cancer only

8. Comprehensive documentation in oncology coding is necessary to support:

A. The use of luxury facilities

B. Coding of the diagnosis, treatment plan, and administration of therapies

C. The preferences for treatment times

D. The social history of the patient

9. A strategy to overcome challenges in oncology coding does NOT include:

A. Ignoring updates to coding guidelines

B. Collaboration with healthcare providers

C. Utilization of specialized resources

D. Regular auditing and quality checks

10. The coding of hematology treatments focuses on:

A. The age of the patient

B. The administration of blood products and treatments for blood disorders

C. The number of hospital visits

D. The patient's family history of blood disorders

Answers

1. D. HCPCS Level II

2. B. The type, location, and behavior of the neoplasm

3. C. Identifying specific chemotherapy drugs

4. B. Staying updated with coding guidelines and regulations

5. B. Specific circumstances of the care provided

6. B. Staying informed about new treatment modalities and coding updates

7. B. CPT codes for treatment planning, delivery, and management

8. B. Coding of the diagnosis, treatment plan, and administration of therapies

9. A. Ignoring updates to coding guidelines

10. B. The administration of blood products and treatments for blood disorders

Chapter 19: Quality and Audit in Medical Coding

19.1. Importance of Coding Quality

The quality of medical coding within healthcare organizations is paramount, influencing not only financial reimbursement but also patient care, data reporting, and compliance with healthcare regulations. High-quality coding practices ensure accurate representation of patient encounters, facilitating effective communication among healthcare providers, payers, and regulatory bodies.

Key Aspects Highlighting the Importance of Coding Quality

1. Accurate Reimbursement:

- Quality coding directly impacts the financial health of healthcare providers by ensuring accurate billing and maximizing reimbursement. Precise coding minimizes claim denials and rejections due to coding errors, streamlining the revenue cycle process.

2. Compliance with Regulations and Standards:

- Adherence to coding guidelines and standards is crucial for compliance with federal and state regulations, including those related to the Health Insurance Portability and Accountability Act (HIPAA) and the Centers for Medicare & Medicaid Services (CMS). Quality coding practices reduce the risk of audits and penalties associated with non-compliance.

3. Enhanced Patient Care:

- Accurate coding provides a detailed and accurate medical record, which is essential for effective patient care management. It ensures that healthcare providers have access to comprehensive patient information, supporting clinical decision-making and continuity of care.

4. Reliable Data for Reporting and Analysis:

- High-quality coding contributes to the reliability of healthcare data, which is used for a variety of purposes, including public health reporting, healthcare policy development, and clinical research. Accurate data supports efforts to improve healthcare quality, patient outcomes, and population health management.

5. Benchmarking and Performance Improvement:

- Quality coding allows healthcare organizations to benchmark their performance against industry standards and identify areas for improvement. It supports quality assurance and performance improvement initiatives aimed at enhancing healthcare delivery and patient satisfaction.

Strategies to Enhance Coding Quality

1. Continuous Education and Training:

- Provide ongoing education and training for coding staff on the latest coding guidelines, regulatory requirements, and best practices to ensure their skills remain current.

2. Implement Coding Audits and Feedback:

- Conduct regular coding audits to assess accuracy and compliance, and provide constructive feedback to coders based on audit findings. Audits help identify areas for improvement and reinforce high-quality coding practices.

3. Leverage Technology and Coding Tools:

- Utilize advanced coding software and tools that incorporate current coding guidelines and offer features such as code validation and error checking to support quality coding.

4. Foster Collaboration Among Coding and Clinical Staff:

- Encourage open communication and collaboration between coding professionals and clinical staff to clarify documentation and ensure accurate code assignment. This collaboration enhances the quality of both coding and clinical documentation.

5. Develop and Enforce Coding Policies and Procedures:

- Establish clear coding policies and procedures that align with industry standards and regulatory requirements. Regularly review and update these policies to reflect changes in coding practices and regulations.

Conclusion

The importance of coding quality in the healthcare industry cannot be overstated, as it underpins financial viability, regulatory compliance, patient care, and the integrity of healthcare data. By adopting comprehensive strategies to maintain and improve coding quality, healthcare organizations can ensure accurate documentation and coding of patient encounters, supporting their overall mission and objectives.

19.2. Conducting Coding Audits

Conducting coding audits is a crucial aspect of maintaining high coding quality within healthcare organizations. Audits not only ensure compliance with coding standards and regulations but also identify opportunities for improvement in coding practices, thereby enhancing revenue integrity and supporting patient care.

Purpose of Coding Audits

1. **Compliance Assurance:** Verify adherence to current coding guidelines, payer policies, and regulatory requirements to minimize the risk of non-compliance and associated penalties.

2. **Revenue Optimization:** Identify undercoding or overcoding instances to ensure accurate reimbursement for services rendered, preventing revenue loss or the risk of fraudulent billing.

3. **Educational Feedback:** Provide coders with constructive feedback based on audit findings, highlighting areas for improvement and reinforcing correct coding practices.

4. **Data Quality Improvement:** Enhance the accuracy of coded data used for reporting, decision-making, and healthcare analytics, contributing to better healthcare outcomes and strategic planning.

5. **Risk Management:** Identify and mitigate potential risks related to coding practices, including those that could lead to claim denials, audits by external entities, or legal challenges.

Types of Coding Audits

1. **Prospective Audits:** Conducted before claims are submitted to payers, allowing for corrections in real-time and reducing the risk of claim rejections or denials.

2. **Retrospective Audits:** Performed after claims have been processed and reimbursed, focusing on identifying trends, areas of risk, and opportunities for education.

3. **Random Audits:** Involves selecting a random sample of claims for review, providing a general overview of coding accuracy and compliance.

4. **Targeted Audits:** Focuses on specific areas of concern, such as high-risk services, specialties with historically high error rates, or services frequently audited by external agencies.

Steps in Conducting a Coding Audit

1. **Planning:** Define the scope, objectives, and methodology of the audit. Determine the sample size and selection criteria for the records to be audited.

2. **Execution:** Review the selected records, comparing documented services with coded items. Assess adherence to coding guidelines and the accuracy of code assignment.

3. **Analysis:** Compile audit findings, identifying patterns of errors, discrepancies, and areas of non-compliance. Calculate the accuracy rate and the potential financial impact of identified coding issues.

4. **Reporting:** Prepare a comprehensive audit report summarizing the findings, including specific examples of coding inaccuracies, areas of risk, and recommendations for improvement.

5. **Education and Feedback:** Share the audit results with coding staff, providing targeted education and feedback to address identified issues and reinforce correct coding practices.

6. **Action Plan:** Develop an action plan to address audit findings, including corrective actions, process improvements, and strategies to prevent future coding errors.

Best Practices for Effective Coding Audits

- **Ensure Auditor Expertise:** Auditors should have a thorough understanding of coding guidelines, payer policies, and clinical knowledge relevant to the services audited.

- **Maintain Transparency:** Clearly communicate the purpose, process, and outcomes of audits to coding staff to foster a constructive and educational approach.

- **Follow Up:** Monitor the implementation of corrective actions and the effectiveness of educational interventions through subsequent audits or quality checks.

- **Foster a Culture of Continuous Improvement:** Encourage an organizational culture that views audits as opportunities for learning and improvement rather than punitive measures.

Conclusion

Coding audits are an integral component of a comprehensive coding quality and compliance program. By systematically reviewing coding practices and providing feedback, healthcare organizations can enhance coding accuracy, ensure compliance, optimize revenue, and ultimately support high-quality patient care.

19.3. Addressing Common Coding Errors

Identifying and addressing common coding errors is crucial for maintaining the integrity of medical billing and coding processes. These errors can lead to claim denials, compliance issues, and financial losses for healthcare organizations. By understanding frequent mistakes and implementing strategies to prevent them, coding quality can be significantly improved.

Common Coding Errors

1. **Incorrect Use of Modifiers:** Misapplying modifiers or failing to use them when necessary can lead to inaccurate billing and claim denials.

2. **Upcoding and Undercoding:** Upcoding (coding for a higher level of service than provided) and undercoding (not coding to the full extent of services provided) can result from misunderstanding documentation or an attempt to avoid audits, both of which have compliance implications.

3. **Lack of Specificity in Diagnosis Coding:** Not using the most specific codes available in ICD-10-CM can result in denied claims or requests for additional information, delaying reimbursement.

4. **Mismatch Between Procedure Codes and Diagnosis Codes:** The procedure codes must accurately reflect the diagnosis codes to establish medical necessity. Mismatches can lead to claim denials.

5. **Unbundling:** Coding individual components of a procedure that should be reported with a comprehensive code leads to unbundling errors, potentially resulting in overpayment demands during audits.

6. **Duplicate Billing:** Submitting multiple claims for a service that should only be billed once can occur due to clerical errors or misunderstanding of billing guidelines.

Strategies to Address Coding Errors

1. **Continuous Education and Training:** Regularly update coding staff on the latest coding guidelines, changes in payer policies, and common coding pitfalls to keep their skills sharp and reduce errors.

2. **Use of Coding Audits:** Implement both prospective and retrospective coding audits to identify and address errors before claims submission and to learn from past mistakes, respectively.

3. **Clear Documentation Guidelines:** Ensure that healthcare providers understand the importance of detailed and specific documentation to support accurate coding and establish medical necessity.

4. **Regular Feedback and Communication:** Provide coding staff with feedback on their coding accuracy and create channels for coders to ask questions or seek clarification from providers to prevent errors.

5. **Leveraging Technology:** Utilize advanced coding software and electronic health record (EHR) systems that include built-in checks for coding accuracy, such as alerts for potential unbundling or mismatched codes.

6. **Development of a Coding Compliance Plan:** Establish a comprehensive coding compliance plan that includes policies for regular audits, staff education, error reporting, and corrective action processes.

7. **Fostering a Culture of Quality:** Promote a culture that prioritizes coding quality and accuracy over speed, recognizing that preventing errors is more efficient than correcting them after the fact.

Conclusion

Addressing common coding errors is an ongoing challenge that requires a multifaceted approach, including education, technology, and effective communication. By focusing on these areas, healthcare organizations can improve their coding accuracy, reduce the risk of claim denials, and ensure compliance with healthcare regulations, ultimately supporting their financial health and the quality of patient care.

19.4. Strategies for Quality Improvement in Coding

Improving coding quality is essential for healthcare organizations to ensure accurate reimbursement, compliance with regulations, and the integrity of medical records. Implementing effective strategies for quality improvement can lead to significant benefits, including reduced claim denials, enhanced revenue cycle management, and improved patient care documentation.

Key Strategies for Enhancing Coding Quality

1. Continuous Education and Training:

- **Objective:** Keep coding staff updated on the latest coding guidelines, regulatory changes, and clinical developments.

- **Implementation:** Offer regular training sessions, workshops, and access to coding webinars and conferences. Encourage coding certification and provide resources for ongoing professional development.

2. Implementation of Coding Audits:

- **Objective:** Identify coding inaccuracies, assess compliance with coding standards, and uncover areas for improvement.

- **Implementation:** Conduct regular prospective and retrospective audits. Use findings to provide targeted feedback and education to coding staff.

3. Utilization of Advanced Coding Technologies:

- **Objective:** Leverage technology to enhance coding accuracy and efficiency.

- **Implementation:** Invest in coding software that includes error-checking features, automated code suggestions, and integration with electronic health records (EHRs). Utilize natural language processing (NLP) tools to assist in extracting relevant information from clinical documentation.

4. Fostering a Collaborative Environment:

- **Objective:** Enhance communication between coders and healthcare providers to improve documentation quality and coding accuracy.

- **Implementation:** Establish regular meetings or communication channels for coders and clinicians to discuss documentation and coding issues. Implement a query process that allows coders to seek clarification on documentation directly from healthcare providers.

5. Development of a Coding Compliance Plan:

- **Objective:** Ensure adherence to coding guidelines and regulatory requirements to mitigate risk and enhance coding integrity.

- **Implementation:** Create a comprehensive coding compliance plan that outlines policies, procedures, and responsibilities. Include guidelines for handling coding errors, conducting audits, and addressing compliance issues.

6. Encouraging Certification and Specialization:

- **Objective:** Promote a higher level of expertise and specialization among coding staff.

- **Implementation:** Support coders in obtaining certification through recognized coding organizations. Encourage specialization in specific areas of medical coding, such as oncology, cardiology, or orthopedics, to improve coding accuracy in complex clinical areas.

7. Promoting a Culture of Quality and Accountability:

- **Objective:** Create an organizational culture that values high-quality coding and holds individuals accountable for their coding practices.

- **Implementation:** Recognize and reward accurate coding and improvements in coding quality. Incorporate coding accuracy and compliance metrics into performance evaluations.

Conclusion

Improving coding quality is a multifaceted effort that requires commitment from both the coding team and the broader healthcare organization. By investing in education, technology, collaboration, and compliance, organizations can create a solid foundation for high-quality coding practices. These strategies not only support the financial and operational goals of healthcare providers but also contribute to the delivery of high-quality patient care.

19.5. Exercise: 10 MCQs with Answers at the End

Test your knowledge on quality improvement and auditing in medical coding, focusing on the importance of coding quality, conducting coding audits, addressing common coding errors, and strategies for enhancing coding quality. Answers are provided at the end for self-assessment.

Questions

1. What is the primary goal of continuous education and training in medical coding?

   A. To increase the speed of coding

   B. To ensure compliance with the latest coding guidelines

   C. To reduce the need for audits

   D. To eliminate the use of technology in coding

2. Coding audits are conducted to:

   A. Penalize coders for mistakes

   B. Identify areas for improvement and ensure compliance

   C. Decrease the workload of coders

   D. Increase the complexity of coding

3. The use of advanced coding technologies aims to:

   A. Replace human coders

   B. Enhance coding accuracy and efficiency

   C. Simplify medical documentation

D. Increase healthcare costs

4. A collaborative environment between coders and healthcare providers helps to:

A. Reduce the importance of coding in healthcare

B. Improve documentation quality and coding accuracy

C. Discourage communication within the healthcare team

D. Focus solely on financial outcomes

5. A coding compliance plan is important for:

A. Ignoring regulatory requirements

B. Ensuring adherence to coding guidelines and reducing risk

C. Limiting coders' access to resources

D. Decreasing organizational transparency

6. Certification and specialization among coding staff:

A. Decrease coding quality

B. Are unnecessary for coding professionals

C. Promote a higher level of expertise and accuracy

D. Are discouraged in the coding profession

7. The primary objective of promoting a culture of quality and accountability is to:

A. Create unnecessary competition among coders

B. Value high-quality coding and hold individuals accountable

C. Eliminate the need for coding audits

D. Reduce collaboration between coders and healthcare providers

8. Common coding errors include all the following EXCEPT:

A. Incorrect use of modifiers

B. Always using the most specific diagnosis codes available

C. Mismatch between procedure codes and diagnosis codes

D. Duplicate billing

9. Effective strategies for coding quality improvement do NOT include:

A. Decreasing education and training opportunities

B. Conducting regular coding audits

C. Utilizing advanced coding technologies

D. Encouraging certification and specialization

10. The main benefit of a collaborative environment in coding is to:

A. Isolate coders from the rest of the healthcare team

B. Ensure that healthcare providers understand coding challenges

C. Improve the accuracy and completeness of clinical documentation

D. Focus on the financial aspects of healthcare only

Answers

1. B. To ensure compliance with the latest coding guidelines

2. B. Identify areas for improvement and ensure compliance

3. B. Enhance coding accuracy and efficiency

4. B. Improve documentation quality and coding accuracy

5. B. Ensuring adherence to coding guidelines and reducing risk

6. C. Promote a higher level of expertise and accuracy

7. B. Value high-quality coding and hold individuals accountable

8. B. Always using the most specific diagnosis codes available

9. A. Decreasing education and training opportunities

10. C. Improve the accuracy and completeness of clinical documentation

Chapter 20: Technology in Medical Coding

20.1. Software Tools for Coders

The integration of technology in medical coding has revolutionized the way coding professionals work, enhancing accuracy, efficiency, and compliance. Software tools specifically designed for coders play a pivotal role in navigating the complexities of medical coding, managing large volumes of data, and ensuring adherence to constantly evolving coding guidelines and regulations.

Key Software Tools for Coders

1. Electronic Health Records (EHR) Systems:

- **Purpose:** EHR systems centralize patient medical records, providing coders with access to comprehensive clinical documentation necessary for accurate code assignment.

- **Features:** Integration with coding software, real-time access to patient data, and documentation tools that support detailed clinical narratives.

2. Computer-Assisted Coding (CAC) Systems:

- **Purpose:** CAC systems use natural language processing (NLP) to automatically identify and extract relevant information from clinical documentation, suggesting appropriate codes for review and validation by coders.

- **Features:** Automated code suggestions, reduction in manual coding time, and support for both ICD-10-CM/PCS and CPT coding.

3. Coding and Billing Software:

- **Purpose:** These tools streamline the coding and billing process, facilitating the submission of claims, management of denials, and tracking of reimbursements.

- **Features:** Claims processing, denial management, and financial reporting capabilities. Integration with payer portals for real-time claim status and eligibility verification.

4. Encoder Software:

- **Purpose:** Encoders provide coders with access to current coding guidelines, code lookup tools, and resources for validating code selections.

- **Features:** Comprehensive code databases, search functionality for quick code lookup, and updates on coding guidelines and payer policies.

5. Audit Software:

- **Purpose:** Audit software supports the quality assurance process by identifying coding inconsistencies, potential compliance issues, and areas for improvement.

- **Features:** Automated coding audits, reporting tools for analyzing audit results, and trend analysis to identify recurring coding issues.

Benefits of Using Software Tools in Medical Coding

- **Increased Accuracy:** Technology helps reduce human errors by providing coders with the latest coding guidelines, automated suggestions, and tools for code verification.

- **Efficiency Gains:** Automated processes and centralized information systems streamline coding tasks, allowing coders to handle higher volumes of work with greater speed.

- **Compliance Support:** Software tools are regularly updated to reflect changes in coding standards and healthcare regulations, aiding in compliance efforts.

- **Data Analytics:** Advanced analytics features offer insights into coding trends, reimbursement patterns, and opportunities for process optimization.

- **Enhanced Collaboration:** Integrated systems facilitate communication between coders, billers, and healthcare providers, ensuring a coordinated approach to patient billing and care documentation.

Considerations When Selecting Coding Software

- **Compatibility:** Ensure the software integrates seamlessly with existing EHR and practice management systems.

- **Usability:** Look for user-friendly interfaces that support efficient workflow and ease of use.

- **Support and Training:** Consider the level of customer support and training resources provided to maximize the benefits of the software.

- **Security:** Assess the software's security features to ensure patient data is protected in compliance with HIPAA and other privacy regulations.

Conclusion

Software tools are indispensable in modern medical coding, offering solutions that enhance the accuracy, efficiency, and compliance of coding practices. By leveraging these technologies, coding professionals can better navigate the complexities of medical documentation and coding guidelines, contributing to the overall success and sustainability of healthcare organizations.

20.2. Leveraging Coding Databases and Resources

In the dynamic field of medical coding, staying informed about the latest coding guidelines, updates, and best practices is crucial. Coding databases and online resources play a vital role in providing coders with the necessary tools to ensure accuracy, compliance, and efficiency in their work.

Key Coding Databases and Resources

1. ICD-10-CM and ICD-10-PCS Online Databases:

- **Purpose:** Offer comprehensive information on diagnosis and procedure codes, including detailed descriptions, coding guidelines, and instructional notes.

- **Features:** Searchable databases, official coding guidelines, and annual updates to codes and guidelines.

2. CPT® Assistant and HCPCS Level II Online Resources:

- **Purpose:** Provide guidance on the correct application of CPT and HCPCS Level II codes, including clarifications on complex coding scenarios and changes to coding rules.

- **Features:** Articles, coding tips, and FAQs authored by the American Medical Association (AMA) and CMS, offering insights into procedural coding.

3. Encoder Software and Online Coding Tools:

- **Purpose:** Assist coders in finding the correct codes quickly and verifying coding decisions against current guidelines and payer policies.

- **Features:** Code lookup tools, cross-reference capabilities, and updates on coding changes.

4. Professional Coding Forums and Discussion Boards:

- **Purpose:** Facilitate knowledge sharing and problem-solving among coding professionals.

- **Features:** Platforms for asking coding-related questions, sharing experiences, and discussing challenges with peers.

5. CMS and Specialty Society Websites:

- **Purpose:** Provide official coding guidelines, policy updates, and educational materials specific to various medical specialties.

- **Features:** Regulatory updates, coding policy manuals, and specialty-specific coding advice.

6. Coding Webinars and Online Training Platforms:

- **Purpose:** Offer ongoing education on coding topics, including updates to coding systems, compliance issues, and coding for specific medical conditions or treatments.

- **Features:** Live and on-demand webinars, online courses, and certification preparation materials.

Benefits of Leveraging Coding Databases and Resources

- **Enhanced Accuracy:** Access to authoritative coding information and guidelines supports precise code assignment, reducing errors and claim denials.

- **Up-to-Date Knowledge:** Regular updates on coding changes and healthcare regulations ensure coders stay informed about the latest developments in their field.

- **Increased Efficiency:** Online tools and databases allow for quick code lookup and verification, streamlining the coding process.

- **Professional Development:** Educational resources and forums support the continuous learning and professional growth of coding staff.

- **Compliance Support:** Detailed guidelines and policy information aid in maintaining compliance with coding standards and payer requirements.

Strategies for Effective Use of Coding Databases and Resources

- **Regular Review:** Schedule time regularly to review updates and new information on trusted coding databases and websites.

- **Active Participation:** Engage in coding forums and discussion boards to share knowledge and learn from the experiences of fellow coders.

- **Continuing Education:** Take advantage of webinars, online courses, and training programs to enhance coding skills and knowledge.

- **Bookmarking Key Resources:** Create a curated list of frequently used resources for quick access to important coding information.

- **Collaboration:** Share useful resources and information with coding colleagues to foster a culture of continuous improvement and learning.

Conclusion

Coding databases and online resources are invaluable assets for medical coders, providing the knowledge and tools needed to navigate the complexities of coding accurately and efficiently. By actively leveraging these resources, coders can enhance their coding practices, contribute to the financial and operational success of healthcare organizations, and support the delivery of high-quality patient care.

20.3. Impact of Artificial Intelligence on Coding

Artificial Intelligence (AI) is transforming medical coding, offering unprecedented opportunities to improve accuracy, efficiency, and compliance. By leveraging AI technologies, healthcare organizations can navigate the complexities of coding guidelines and payer policies more effectively, ensuring that medical services are coded correctly and reimbursed appropriately.

Key AI Technologies in Medical Coding

1. Natural Language Processing (NLP):

- **Purpose:** NLP technologies interpret and extract relevant information from unstructured clinical documentation, identifying diagnoses, procedures, and other pertinent details for coding.

- **Impact:** Enhances the accuracy of code assignment by analyzing clinical narratives and suggesting appropriate codes, reducing the reliance on manual coding processes.

2. Machine Learning Algorithms:

- **Purpose:** Machine learning models learn from vast datasets of coded medical records, continuously improving their ability to predict accurate codes based on documentation.

- **Impact:** Increases coding efficiency by automating the coding process for routine cases, allowing coders to focus on more complex scenarios that require human expertise.

3. Predictive Analytics:

- **Purpose:** Uses historical data to predict coding trends, potential errors, and areas of risk before they become significant issues.

- **Impact:** Supports proactive compliance and quality assurance efforts, identifying patterns that could lead to denials or audits and suggesting corrective actions.

Benefits of AI in Medical Coding

- **Reduced Coding Errors:** AI technologies help minimize human errors by providing code suggestions based on the analysis of clinical documentation and coding guidelines.

- **Improved Productivity:** Automating routine coding tasks allows coding professionals to concentrate on complex cases, enhancing overall productivity and job satisfaction.

- **Enhanced Revenue Integrity:** Accurate and efficient coding driven by AI technologies ensures that healthcare providers are reimbursed correctly for the services they deliver, optimizing revenue cycles.

- **Compliance and Audit Readiness:** AI-driven analytics can identify potential compliance issues and audit risks, facilitating corrective measures and improving audit outcomes.

- **Data-Driven Decision Making:** The use of AI in coding generates valuable insights into coding practices, healthcare trends, and operational efficiencies, informing strategic decisions.

Challenges and Considerations

- **Data Privacy and Security:** Implementing AI in coding requires careful consideration of patient data privacy and adherence to regulations such as HIPAA.

- **Integration with Existing Systems:** Seamless integration of AI technologies with current EHR and coding systems is essential for maximizing benefits and minimizing disruptions.

- **Training and Adaptation:** Coders and healthcare professionals need training to work effectively with AI tools, including understanding their capabilities and limitations.

- **Ongoing Monitoring and Evaluation:** AI systems require continuous monitoring to ensure their accuracy and relevance, with periodic evaluations to adjust algorithms based on changing coding guidelines and clinical practices.

Future Directions

The future of AI in medical coding looks promising, with ongoing advancements expected to further refine AI capabilities. As AI technologies become more sophisticated, they will play an increasingly integral role in coding workflows, enhancing precision and efficiency while supporting the transition towards more proactive and strategic coding practices.

Conclusion

AI's impact on medical coding is profound, offering the potential to revolutionize how coding is performed. By embracing AI technologies, healthcare organizations can improve coding quality, streamline operations, and ensure financial sustainability, all while maintaining high standards of patient care and compliance.

20.4. Future Trends in Medical Coding Technology

The landscape of medical coding is continuously evolving, with technology playing a pivotal role in shaping its future. Emerging trends in medical coding technology are set to address current challenges, enhance coding accuracy and efficiency, and support the overall goals of healthcare organizations. Here's a look at some key future trends in medical coding technology.

Integration of Artificial Intelligence and Machine Learning

- **Overview:** The integration of AI and machine learning technologies into medical coding processes is expected to become more sophisticated. These technologies can analyze vast amounts of data to predict accurate codes, identify patterns that may lead to denials, and suggest improvements in coding practices.

- **Impact:** Enhanced productivity and accuracy, reduced denial rates, and improved compliance with coding standards.

Advanced Natural Language Processing (NLP)

- **Overview:** NLP technologies will advance to better understand and interpret the nuances of clinical documentation, extracting relevant information more accurately for coding purposes.

- **Impact:** Increased automation of coding tasks, reduced dependency on manual coding, and the ability to focus human expertise on complex coding scenarios.

Blockchain for Data Security and Integrity

- **Overview:** Blockchain technology offers a secure and transparent way to manage healthcare data, including medical coding information. It can ensure the integrity of coding data and facilitate secure sharing between entities.

- **Impact:** Enhanced data security, improved trust in coding data, and streamlined audits and compliance checks.

Predictive Analytics for Proactive Coding Management

- **Overview:** Predictive analytics will play a larger role in foreseeing coding trends and potential issues before they arise, allowing healthcare organizations to be proactive rather than reactive.

- **Impact:** Prevention of coding errors, anticipation of payer denials, and strategic planning for coding department resources.

Increased Use of Cloud-Based Coding Platforms

- **Overview:** Cloud-based coding platforms allow for real-time updates, collaboration, and access to coding resources from anywhere, facilitating remote work and ensuring coders have the most current information.

- **Impact:** Greater flexibility, scalability, and collaboration among coding teams, along with enhanced access to up-to-date coding guidelines and resources.

Greater Emphasis on Coding Education and Certification Platforms

- **Overview:** As coding becomes more complex, there will be an increased emphasis on continuous education and certification for coders. Online platforms offering specialized coding education and certification will become more prevalent.

- **Impact:** Coders will have greater opportunities for professional development, ensuring they remain proficient in the latest coding practices and technologies.

Patient-Centric Coding Approaches

- **Overview:** Future technologies will enable more patient-centric coding approaches, integrating patient feedback and outcomes into the coding process to better reflect the quality of care provided.

- **Impact:** Improved accuracy in coding for outcomes and patient satisfaction, influencing reimbursement models focused on value-based care.

Conclusion

The future of medical coding technology is bright, with advancements aimed at improving the efficiency, accuracy, and security of coding processes. As these technologies continue to evolve, coders and healthcare organizations must adapt to leverage these innovations effectively, ensuring they meet the demands of modern healthcare delivery and reimbursement models while maintaining high standards of patient care.

20.5. Exercise: 10 MCQs with Answers at the End

Test your knowledge on the future trends and technology in medical coding, covering software tools for coders, leveraging coding databases and resources, the impact of artificial intelligence on coding, and future trends in medical coding technology. Answers are provided at the end for self-assessment.

Questions

1. What technology is primarily used to interpret and extract relevant information from clinical documentation for coding purposes?

   A. Blockchain

   B. Natural Language Processing (NLP)

   C. Cloud Computing

   D. Predictive Analytics

2. Machine learning in medical coding is used to:

   A. Replace human coders entirely

   B. Predict accurate codes based on data patterns

   C. Store patient records securely

   D. Simplify healthcare regulations

3. The use of blockchain technology in medical coding could improve:

   A. Coding speed

   B. Data security and integrity

C. The accuracy of predictive analytics

D. Natural language processing capabilities

4. Predictive analytics in medical coding helps to:

A. Create more complex coding guidelines

B. Foresee coding trends and potential issues

C. Decrease the need for coding audits

D. Increase manual coding tasks

5. Cloud-based coding platforms offer benefits such as:

A. Reduced need for data security

B. Limited access to coding resources

C. Real-time updates and collaboration

D. Complete automation of the coding process

6. Continuous education and certification for coders are becoming more important due to:

A. Decreasing complexity in medical coding

B. The static nature of coding guidelines

C. Advances in coding technology and practices

D. The reduced role of coding in healthcare

7. Artificial Intelligence (AI) impacts medical coding by:

   A. Decreasing coding accuracy over time

   B. Enhancing productivity and accuracy

   C. Eliminating the need for coders' expertise

   D. Making coding guidelines less important

8. Advanced NLP technologies in coding aim to:

   A. Reduce the amount of clinical documentation

   B. Replace predictive analytics

   C. Better understand and interpret clinical documentation

   D. Focus solely on blockchain integration

9. The future trend of patient-centric coding approaches in medical coding is expected to:

   A. Decrease the relevance of patient feedback

   B. Integrate patient outcomes into the coding process

   C. Simplify coding guidelines significantly

   D. Focus coding practices exclusively on reimbursement

10. The main reason for leveraging coding databases and online resources is to:

A. Reduce the interaction between coders and healthcare providers

B. Ensure coders are informed about the latest developments and guidelines

C. Completely automate the coding process

D. Focus coding on administrative tasks only

Answers

1. B. Natural Language Processing (NLP)

2. B. Predict accurate codes based on data patterns

3. B. Data security and integrity

4. B. Foresee coding trends and potential issues

5. C. Real-time updates and collaboration

6. C. Advances in coding technology and practices

7. B. Enhancing productivity and accuracy

8. C. Better understand and interpret clinical documentation

9. B. Integrate patient outcomes into the coding process

10. B. Ensure coders are informed about the latest developments and guidelines

Chapter 21: Professional Development and Certification

21.1. Preparing for Coding Certification

Earning a certification in medical coding is a crucial step for professionals looking to advance their careers, demonstrate their expertise, and stand out in the healthcare industry. Coding certifications validate a coder's knowledge of coding guidelines, medical terminology, anatomy, and the ability to apply this knowledge in practical settings.

Key Coding Certifications

- **Certified Professional Coder (CPC)** offered by the American Academy of Professional Coders (AAPC).

- **Certified Coding Specialist (CCS)** offered by the American Health Information Management Association (AHIMA).

- **Certified Coding Associate (CCA)** also offered by AHIMA, considered an entry-level certification.

Steps to Prepare for Coding Certification

1. Understand Certification Requirements:

- Review the specific requirements for the certification you are pursuing, including education prerequisites, examination topics, and any experience requirements.

2. Enroll in a Coding Education Program:

- Consider enrolling in a coding education program accredited by a recognized body. These programs cover essential topics like medical terminology, anatomy, coding systems (ICD-10-CM/PCS, CPT, HCPCS), and healthcare laws.

3. Gain Practical Experience:

- Practical coding experience is invaluable. If you're new to coding, consider internships, volunteer work, or entry-level positions in medical coding to gain hands-on experience.

4. Use Study Guides and Practice Exams:

- Utilize study guides and practice exams provided by the certifying organizations. These resources are tailored to the exam content and can help identify areas where further study is needed.

5. Join Study Groups:

- Participating in study groups can provide support, clarification of difficult concepts, and exposure to a variety of coding scenarios.

6. Schedule Regular Study Time:

- Consistent study is key. Set aside regular study time in a distraction-free environment to cover the material and practice coding cases.

7. Stay Updated on Coding Guidelines:

- Coding guidelines and regulations change regularly. Stay informed on the latest updates through professional organizations, webinars, and industry publications.

8. Take Care of Logistics Early:

- Register for the exam well in advance, familiarize yourself with the testing location, and ensure you have all necessary materials and identification on exam day.

After Earning Your Certification

- **Maintain Certification:** Most certifications require continuing education units (CEUs) to maintain active status. Engage in ongoing learning and professional development opportunities to meet these requirements.

- **Network with Professionals:** Join professional organizations, attend conferences, and connect with peers in the field to share knowledge and stay informed about industry trends.

- **Explore Career Advancements:** Certification can open doors to new job opportunities, specializations, and leadership roles within healthcare organizations.

Conclusion

Preparing for coding certification requires dedication, study, and practical experience. Achieving certification is a significant milestone in a coder's professional development, offering numerous benefits in terms of career advancement, recognition, and personal satisfaction. By following a structured preparation plan and staying committed to ongoing learning, aspiring coders can achieve success in their certification exams and future careers in medical coding.

21.2. Continuing Education for Medical Coders

Continuing education is a cornerstone of professional development for medical coders. Given the ever-evolving landscape of healthcare regulations, coding guidelines, and medical practices, continuous learning is essential to maintain coding accuracy, compliance, and efficiency. It ensures coders stay updated on the latest developments in their field, ultimately supporting their career growth and the quality of healthcare administration.

Importance of Continuing Education

- **Maintaining Certification:** Many coding certifications require coders to earn continuing education units (CEUs) to keep their credentials active.

- **Adapting to Changes:** Healthcare coding standards, such as ICD, CPT, and HCPCS codes, are regularly updated. Continuous education helps coders adapt to these changes.

- **Enhancing Professional Competence:** Ongoing education broadens a coder's knowledge base, enhancing their coding skills and professional competence.

- **Compliance and Accuracy:** Staying informed about the latest regulations and coding practices helps prevent coding errors and compliance issues.

Sources of Continuing Education

1. Professional Organizations:

- Organizations like the American Academy of Professional Coders (AAPC) and the American Health Information Management Association (AHIMA) offer a wealth of continuing education opportunities, including webinars, workshops, conferences, and online courses.

2. Online Courses and Webinars:

- Numerous platforms provide online courses and webinars covering various topics relevant to medical coding, billing, compliance, and healthcare management.

3. Coding Conferences and Seminars:

- National and regional coding conferences and seminars offer opportunities to learn from industry experts, network with peers, and earn CEUs.

4. College and University Courses:

- Many academic institutions offer courses in medical coding, healthcare administration, and related fields that can count toward continuing education requirements.

5. Industry Publications and Journals:

- Reading industry publications, coding manuals updates, and professional journals is an excellent way to stay informed and may also earn coders CEUs.

Strategies for Effective Continuing Education

1. Plan Ahead:

- Keep track of CEU requirements and deadlines for your certification(s). Plan your continuing education activities to ensure you meet these requirements on time.

2. Diversify Learning Activities:

- Engage in a variety of learning activities to cover different areas of interest and expertise, such as coding practices, compliance, healthcare technology, and management skills.

3. Leverage Technology:

- Utilize online platforms and technology to access educational content and complete coursework conveniently, especially if balancing work and learning.

4. Apply New Knowledge:

- Seek opportunities to apply what you've learned in your work to reinforce new concepts and demonstrate the value of your continuing education efforts.

5. Network and Collaborate:

- Participate in study groups, professional forums, and networking events to share knowledge, discuss industry trends, and learn from the experiences of fellow coders.

Conclusion

Continuing education is indispensable for medical coders committed to excellence in their profession. By actively engaging in learning opportunities and staying abreast of industry developments, coders can ensure they provide the highest level of coding accuracy and integrity, benefiting their careers and the healthcare organizations they serve.

21.3. Networking and Professional Organizations

Networking and involvement in professional organizations are vital aspects of career development for medical coders. These activities offer opportunities for continuing education, staying updated on industry trends, and connecting with peers and experts in the field. Active participation in professional networks can lead to career advancement, enhanced knowledge, and a broader understanding of the healthcare industry's challenges and opportunities.

Benefits of Networking and Professional Organizations

1. Educational Resources and Continuing Education:

- Access to a wide range of educational materials, webinars, workshops, and conferences that contribute to professional growth and fulfill continuing education requirements.

2. Certification and Specialization Opportunities:

- Information and guidance on obtaining certifications and specializations that enhance credibility and expertise in medical coding.

3. Industry Updates and Regulatory Changes:

- Timely updates on coding guidelines, healthcare regulations, and policy changes, ensuring that professionals remain compliant and informed.

4. Career Development and Job Opportunities:

- Networking can lead to job opportunities, mentorship, and career advice from experienced professionals in the field.

5. Advocacy and Representation:

- Professional organizations often advocate on behalf of their members for industry standards, fair practices, and policies that impact the medical coding profession.

6. Peer Support and Community:

- A sense of community and support from peers facing similar challenges and goals in the medical coding field.

Key Professional Organizations for Medical Coders

1. American Academy of Professional Coders (AAPC):

- Offers certification, continuing education, and networking opportunities for medical coders, billers, auditors, and compliance officers.

2. American Health Information Management Association (AHIMA):

- Provides resources for health information management professionals, including coders, with a focus on data quality and privacy, certification, and education.

3. Healthcare Financial Management Association (HFMA):

- While broader in scope, HFMA offers resources and networking opportunities relevant to the financial aspects of healthcare, including medical coding and billing.

Strategies for Effective Networking

1. Attend Industry Conferences and Seminars:

- Participate in national and regional conferences to learn from industry experts and meet fellow professionals.

2. Join Local Chapters and Study Groups:

- Engage with local chapters of professional organizations and participate in study groups to share knowledge and experiences.

3. Utilize Online Forums and Social Media:

- Participate in online forums, LinkedIn groups, and other social media platforms dedicated to medical coding and health information management.

4. Volunteer for Committees or Projects:

- Get involved in committees or projects within professional organizations to contribute your skills and gain visibility in the community.

5. Mentorship:

- Seek out mentorship opportunities or offer to mentor newcomers to the field, fostering professional growth and development for both parties.

Conclusion

Networking and active involvement in professional organizations are crucial for the career advancement of medical coders. These activities offer invaluable resources for education, certification, career development, and staying informed about the ever-changing landscape of healthcare coding and regulation. By leveraging these opportunities, medical coders can enhance their professional skills, contribute to the field, and build a supportive network of colleagues and mentors.

21.4. Career Advancement in Medical Coding

Career advancement in medical coding offers numerous pathways for professionals seeking to elevate their expertise, responsibilities, and earning potential. Advancement can be achieved through specialization, certification, education, and taking on leadership roles. As the healthcare industry continues to evolve, the demand for skilled coding professionals with advanced knowledge and leadership abilities grows.

Paths to Career Advancement

1. Specialization:

- **Overview:** Specializing in a specific area of medical coding, such as oncology, cardiology, or orthopedics, can make coders more valuable to employers and increase their marketability.

- **Approach:** Obtain certifications specific to your area of interest and gain experience in that specialty.

2. Additional Certifications:

- **Overview:** Earning advanced certifications, such as Certified Professional Coder (CPC), Certified Coding Specialist (CCS), or

Certified Inpatient Coder (CIC), demonstrates a higher level of expertise.

- **Approach:** Pursue continuing education and prepare for certification exams that align with your career goals.

3. Leadership Roles:

- **Overview:** Moving into supervisory or management positions, such as coding manager, compliance officer, or HIM director, requires not only coding expertise but also leadership and management skills.

- **Approach:** Develop leadership skills through training, mentorship, and taking on project leadership or supervisory responsibilities within your current role.

4. Education and Training:

- **Overview:** Engaging in ongoing education and training not only keeps coders up-to-date on the latest coding practices but also opens doors to teaching and training opportunities.

- **Approach:** Consider earning a higher degree in health information management or a related field, and seek opportunities to teach coding courses or workshops.

5. Health Information Technology:

- **Overview:** The integration of technology into healthcare provides opportunities for coders to transition into health information technology roles, focusing on EHR management, coding software development, or data analytics.

- **Approach:** Gain knowledge and experience in health IT systems, data management, and analytics tools.

Strategies for Career Advancement

- **Networking:** Build professional relationships through networking events, professional organizations, and online forums. Networking can lead to mentorship opportunities and insider knowledge about job openings and career advancement paths.

- **Continuing Education:** Stay informed about industry trends, regulatory changes, and advancements in coding practices through webinars, conferences, and certification courses.

- **Performance Excellence:** Demonstrate excellence in your current role by maintaining high coding accuracy, productivity, and compliance. High performance can lead to recognition and advancement opportunities.

- **Professional Visibility:** Contribute to professional publications, speak at industry events, or participate in professional organizations to increase your visibility in the field.

- **Leverage Technology:** Embrace technological advancements in coding and health information management. Being proficient in the latest technology can position you for roles that require tech-savvy professionals.

Conclusion

Career advancement in medical coding requires a combination of specialized knowledge, certification, leadership skills, and a commitment to ongoing education. By strategically pursuing these paths and leveraging opportunities for growth, coding professionals can achieve rewarding careers that contribute significantly to the healthcare industry's efficiency and effectiveness.

21.5. Exercise: 10 MCQs with Answers at the End

Test your understanding of professional development and certification in medical coding, including preparing for coding certification, continuing education, networking, and career advancement. Answers are provided at the end for self-assessment.

Questions

1. What is a primary benefit of obtaining a specialized coding certification?

   A. Decreases the need for continuing education

   B. Limits career options to a narrow field

C. Enhances marketability and potential for higher earnings

D. Simplifies the coding process

2. Continuing education for medical coders is important to:

A. Maintain coding certification and stay updated on industry changes

B. Eliminate the need for coding audits

C. Reduce the complexity of medical coding

D. Decrease collaboration with healthcare providers

3. Participating in professional organizations can provide medical coders with:

A. Less exposure to coding trends and regulations

B. Fewer networking opportunities

C. Access to educational resources and industry updates

D. An increased workload

4. A coder looking to advance their career might pursue:

A. Less responsibility and fewer duties

B. Specialization in an area like oncology or cardiology

C. Avoidance of technology in coding processes

D. Decreased focus on coding accuracy

5. Leadership roles in medical coding require:

   A. Only basic coding knowledge

   B. Leadership and management skills

   C. A preference for working in isolation

   D. No additional certifications

6. Health Information Technology (HIT) roles may appeal to medical coders interested in:

   A. Avoiding coding altogether

   B. Working exclusively with paper records

   C. EHR management and data analytics

   D. Reducing their interaction with healthcare providers

7. Networking is crucial for medical coders because it:

   A. Decreases professional opportunities

   B. Limits access to new information

   C. Can lead to mentorship and job opportunities

   D. Requires less professional development

8. The main reason for coders to engage in continuing education is to:

   A. Focus solely on historical coding practices

   B. Stay informed about the latest coding practices and guidelines

   C. Avoid networking with other professionals

   D. Decrease their value to employers

9. Which strategy is NOT effective for career advancement in medical coding?

   A. Increasing coding errors to learn from mistakes

   B. Gaining specialized certifications

   C. Engaging in leadership training

   D. Participating in professional organizations

10. The role of technology in medical coding is to:

   A. Complicate the coding process

   B. Replace the need for coders entirely

   C. Enhance coding accuracy and efficiency

   D. Limit access to coding resources

Answers

1. C. Enhances marketability and potential for higher earnings

2. A. Maintain coding certification and stay updated on industry changes

3. C. Access to educational resources and industry updates

4. B. Specialization in an area like oncology or cardiology

5. B. Leadership and management skills

6. C. EHR management and data analytics

7. C. Can lead to mentorship and job opportunities

8. B. Stay informed about the latest coding practices and guidelines

9. A. Increasing coding errors to learn from mistakes

10. C. Enhance coding accuracy and efficiency

Chapter 22: Working as a Freelance Medical Coder

22.1. Starting a Freelance Coding Business

Embarking on a freelance medical coding career offers flexibility, the opportunity to choose projects that align with your interests, and the potential for a better work-life balance. However, it requires careful planning, dedication, and the right strategies to succeed. Here's how to start a freelance medical coding business effectively.

Essential Steps to Start a Freelance Coding Business

1. Gain Necessary Experience and Certification:

- **Overview:** Before starting a freelance career, ensure you have the requisite coding experience and any necessary certifications (e.g., CPC, CCS). These credentials enhance your credibility and marketability to potential clients.

- **Action:** If you're new to coding, consider working in a traditional setting first to gain experience and understand the industry's nuances.

2. Develop a Business Plan:

- **Overview:** A clear business plan outlines your business goals, target market, services offered, pricing strategy, and marketing approach.

- **Action:** Identify your niche within medical coding, such as specific medical specialties or types of coding services, and plan how you will attract and retain clients.

3. Legal and Financial Setup:

- **Overview:** Establishing your freelance business legally includes deciding on a business structure (e.g., sole proprietorship, LLC), registering your business, and setting up a business bank account.

- **Action:** Consult with legal and financial advisors to ensure compliance with local regulations and tax laws.

4. Invest in Technology and Resources:

- **Overview:** Reliable coding software, access to up-to-date coding manuals, and a secure, efficient home office setup are crucial for providing professional coding services.

- **Action:** Research and invest in the necessary technology and subscriptions to coding databases and resources.

5. Marketing and Networking:

- **Overview:** Building a client base requires effective marketing and networking. This can include creating a professional website, leveraging social media, attending industry conferences, and joining professional organizations.

- **Action:** Develop a marketing strategy that highlights your expertise, services, and value proposition to potential clients.

6. Continuous Education and Skill Development:

- **Overview:** Staying current with coding guidelines, healthcare regulations, and continuing education is vital for maintaining your expertise and offering high-quality services.

- **Action:** Allocate time and resources for ongoing education, certification renewals, and professional development.

7. Set Clear Policies and Procedures:

- **Overview:** Clear policies on project management, billing, and communication ensure smooth operations and help manage client expectations.

- **Action:** Develop and communicate your policies on project timelines, rates, revisions, and feedback mechanisms from the outset.

Challenges and Solutions for Freelance Medical Coders

- **Challenge:** Finding consistent work and building a stable client base.

- **Solution:** Diversify your services, network extensively, and consider working with medical coding agencies or subcontracting to establish a steady workflow.

- **Challenge:** Keeping up with industry changes and maintaining certifications.

  - **Solution:** Prioritize continuous learning and leverage professional associations for resources and training opportunities.

- **Challenge:** Managing all aspects of the business, from coding to customer service and billing.

  - **Solution:** Use software tools for billing and project management and consider outsourcing non-core tasks as your business grows.

Conclusion

Starting a freelance medical coding business is a promising venture for those seeking flexibility and independence in their careers. Success in this field requires a combination of coding expertise, business acumen, and proactive marketing. By following these steps and preparing for the inherent challenges of freelance work, medical coders can build rewarding and sustainable freelance careers.

22.2. Marketing and Building Clientele

For freelance medical coders, developing a strong client base is essential for achieving long-term success and stability. Effective marketing strategies and networking efforts are crucial for attracting and retaining clients in a competitive landscape. Here's how freelance medical coders can market their services and build a robust clientele.

Strategies for Marketing and Building Clientele

1. Establish a Professional Online Presence:

- **Website:** Create a professional website that showcases your services, certifications, areas of specialization, and contact information. Include testimonials from satisfied clients to build credibility.

- **Social Media:** Utilize social media platforms, such as LinkedIn, to network with industry professionals and share content related to medical coding, demonstrating your expertise.

2. Networking and Professional Associations:

- Join professional associations like AAPC (American Academy of Professional Coders) and AHIMA (American Health Information Management Association). Attend conferences, workshops, and networking events to meet potential clients and learn about the latest industry trends.

3. Utilize Freelance Platforms and Job Boards:

- Platforms such as Upwork, Freelancer, and specialized job boards for healthcare professionals can be valuable sources for finding freelance coding projects. Create a compelling profile highlighting your experience and skills.

4. Offer Free Educational Content:

- Blogging or creating educational videos about medical coding can establish you as an authority in your field. Share insights on coding best practices, changes in coding guidelines, and tips for healthcare providers.

5. Seek Referrals and Testimonials:

- Encourage satisfied clients to refer your services to others and request testimonials that you can feature on your website and marketing materials.

6. Direct Outreach:

- Identify potential clients, such as medical practices, billing companies, and healthcare facilities, and reach out directly with tailored proposals that highlight how your services can benefit them.

7. Leverage Local Community Connections:

- Engage with your local healthcare community, including medical associations and small practices, where there may be a need for freelance coding services.

Tips for Effective Client Communication and Retention

1. Clear Communication:

- Establish clear communication channels and processes. Be responsive to client inquiries and proactive in providing updates on project progress.

2. Quality and Accuracy:

- Ensure the highest quality and accuracy in your coding work. Consistently meeting or exceeding client expectations can lead to repeat business and referrals.

3. Customized Solutions:

- Understand the specific needs of each client and offer customized coding solutions. Personalized service can set you apart from competitors.

4. Professional Development:

- Stay updated on industry standards and regulations to provide clients with the most current and compliant coding services.

5. Follow-up and Feedback:

- After project completion, follow up with clients to ensure their satisfaction and seek feedback on how you can improve your services.

Conclusion

Marketing and building a clientele as a freelance medical coder requires a combination of professional online presence, effective networking, high-quality service delivery, and excellent client communication. By implementing these strategies, freelance coders can establish a sustainable and rewarding career, contributing valuable services to the healthcare industry.

22.3. Managing a Freelance Coding Business

Running a successful freelance medical coding business involves more than just coding expertise. It requires effective business management, including financial planning, client relations, project management, and continuous professional development. Here's how to manage a freelance coding business effectively.

Financial Management

1. Pricing Strategies:

- **Overview:** Set competitive yet profitable pricing for your services based on the complexity of the work, your experience, and market rates. Consider different pricing models, such as hourly rates or project-based fees.

- **Action:** Conduct market research to understand what others in your field charge and adjust your rates accordingly to remain competitive and fair.

2. Financial Tracking and Invoicing:

- **Overview:** Keep accurate records of income and expenses. Use accounting software to track financial transactions, manage invoices, and prepare for tax obligations.

- **Action:** Regularly update financial records and follow up on outstanding invoices to maintain a steady cash flow.

Client Relationship Management

1. Clear Communication and Expectations:

- **Overview:** Establish clear communication channels and set realistic expectations regarding deliverables, timelines, and feedback mechanisms.

- **Action:** Create a client agreement or contract that outlines the scope of work, payment terms, and confidentiality clauses.

2. Quality Assurance:

- **Overview:** Ensure the highest quality of coding to build trust and retain clients. Implement a quality assurance process to review and verify coding accuracy.

- **Action:** Stay updated on coding guidelines and participate in continuing education to enhance your coding skills and knowledge.

Project Management

1. Efficient Workflow:

- **Overview:** Develop an efficient workflow to manage multiple projects effectively. Utilize project management tools to track progress, deadlines, and client communication.

- **Action:** Prioritize tasks based on deadlines and client importance. Use software like Trello, Asana, or Notion to organize projects and tasks.

2. Time Management:

- **Overview:** Effective time management is crucial for meeting client deadlines and managing work-life balance.

- **Action:** Allocate specific time blocks for coding, administrative tasks, and professional development. Avoid overcommitting to projects beyond your capacity.

Professional Development

1. Continuing Education:

- **Overview:** Stay abreast of changes in coding guidelines, healthcare regulations, and technology advancements.

- **Action:** Participate in webinars, workshops, and professional conferences. Earn CEUs to maintain coding certifications.

2. Networking and Collaboration:

- **Overview:** Engage with other professionals in the field through online forums, professional associations, and social media.

- **Action:** Share experiences, seek advice, and collaborate on projects when possible. Networking can lead to new opportunities and insights.

Legal and Ethical Considerations

1. Compliance and Ethics:

- **Overview:** Adhere to ethical coding practices and ensure compliance with healthcare regulations, including HIPAA.

- **Action:** Regularly review compliance guidelines and attend training on healthcare privacy and security regulations.

2. Contractual Agreements:

- **Overview:** Protect your business and interests with clear contractual agreements with clients.

- **Action:** Consider consulting with a legal professional to draft or review contracts to ensure they cover scope of work, payment terms, and confidentiality requirements.

Conclusion

Managing a freelance medical coding business requires a multifaceted approach, focusing on financial health, client satisfaction, efficient project management, and ongoing professional growth. By adopting effective business management practices, freelance coders can build sustainable, rewarding careers while contributing significantly to the healthcare industry.

22.4. Challenges of Freelance Medical Coding

While freelance medical coding offers numerous benefits, including flexibility and the opportunity to work on a variety of projects, it also presents several challenges. Recognizing and addressing these challenges early on can help freelance coders establish a successful and sustainable business.

1. Inconsistent Workflows and Income

- **Challenge:** Freelance coders may experience fluctuating workloads and incomes, making financial stability a concern, especially in the early stages of their freelance career.

- **Strategies:**

 - Diversify your client base to reduce dependency on a single source of income.

 - Establish a financial buffer to manage through periods of reduced work.

 - Engage in ongoing marketing efforts to attract new clients.

2. Isolation and Lack of Support

- **Challenge:** Working independently can lead to feelings of isolation and lack of support, which may impact motivation and productivity.

- **Strategies:**

 - Join professional organizations and online communities to connect with peers.

 - Attend industry conferences and workshops to network and stay engaged with the coding community.

 - Consider coworking spaces or local meetups to reduce isolation.

3. Keeping Up with Industry Changes

- **Challenge:** The medical coding field is constantly evolving, with regular updates to coding standards, healthcare regulations, and technology. Staying current can be challenging for freelancers who manage all aspects of their business.

- **Strategies:**

  - Allocate time for continuing education and professional development.

  - Subscribe to industry publications, attend webinars, and participate in training sessions offered by professional organizations.

  - Utilize social media and professional networks to stay informed about industry trends.

4. Managing Business Operations

- **Challenge:** Freelancers must handle business operations, including marketing, client communication, billing, and compliance, in addition to coding tasks.

- **Strategies:**

  - Use business management and accounting software to streamline operations.

  - Set clear policies for billing, client communication, and project management.

  - Consider outsourcing non-core tasks, such as marketing or accounting, to professionals or services.

5. Ensuring Data Security and Compliance

- **Challenge:** Freelancers must ensure the security of patient data and compliance with regulations like HIPAA, which can be daunting without the support of an IT department.

- **Strategies:**

  - Implement robust data security measures, including encrypted communication, secure data storage, and regular security audits.

  - Stay updated on compliance requirements and best practices for data protection.

  - Consider cybersecurity insurance and legal consultation to mitigate risks.

6. Health Insurance and Benefits

- **Challenge:** Unlike traditional employment, freelancers are responsible for securing their health insurance and do not receive benefits like paid leave or retirement plans.

- **Strategies:**

  - Explore health insurance options through professional organizations, the ACA marketplace, or private insurers.

  - Plan for retirement by setting up an IRA or another retirement savings account.

  - Budget for vacations and sick days as part of your annual financial planning.

Conclusion

Freelance medical coding presents unique challenges that require proactive planning and management. By implementing effective strategies to address these challenges, freelance coders can build successful careers that offer both professional satisfaction and personal flexibility. Networking, continuous learning, and efficient business management are key to overcoming the hurdles of freelance work and thriving in the dynamic field of medical coding.

22.5. Exercise: 10 MCQs with Answers at the End

Test your knowledge on working as a freelance medical coder, including starting a freelance coding business, marketing and building clientele, managing a freelance coding business, and addressing the challenges of freelance medical coding. Answers are provided at the end for self-assessment.

Questions

1. Which certification is beneficial for a freelance medical coder to enhance credibility?

A. CPC

B. MBA

C. RN

D. PhD

2. What is a key strategy for managing fluctuating incomes in freelance medical coding?

A. Increasing prices annually

B. Diversifying client base

C. Working exclusively for one client

D. Avoiding long-term contracts

3. An effective way to combat isolation as a freelance medical coder is to:

A. Work longer hours

B. Join professional organizations

C. Reduce networking efforts

D. Limit social media usage

4. Staying updated with industry changes as a freelancer can be achieved through:

A. Ignoring new coding guidelines

B. Focusing solely on one coding system

C. Attending webinars and continuing education courses

D. Avoiding interaction with other coding professionals

5. For freelance medical coders, managing business operations efficiently can be facilitated by:

   A. Manual record-keeping

   B. Avoiding the use of software tools

   C. Using business management and accounting software

   D. Outsourcing coding tasks only

6. Ensuring data security and compliance in freelance medical coding involves:

   A. Sharing passwords with clients for ease of access

   B. Using encrypted communication and secure data storage

   C. Storing all data on easily accessible cloud services

   D. Sending sensitive information via regular email

7. A major challenge for freelance medical coders is:

   A. Too many client requests to handle

   B. Keeping up with industry changes

   C. Mandatory office hours

   D. Guaranteed annual leave

8. Marketing a freelance coding business effectively can include:

A. Avoiding the use of social media

B. Creating a professional website

C. Waiting for clients to contact you first

D. Keeping achievements and certifications private

9. To build a strong client base, freelance medical coders should:

A. Focus on a narrow specialization with limited demand

B. Offer free services to all new clients

C. Engage in ongoing marketing efforts and networking

D. Refrain from seeking referrals and testimonials

10. Addressing the challenge of health insurance and benefits for freelancers involves:

A. Ignoring health insurance needs

B. Relying on emergency funds for medical expenses

C. Exploring health insurance options through professional organizations

D. Waiting for clients to offer health benefits

Answers

1. A. CPC

2. B. Diversifying client base

3. B. Join professional organizations

4. C. Attending webinars and continuing education courses

5. C. Using business management and accounting software

6. B. Using encrypted communication and secure data storage

7. B. Keeping up with industry changes

8. B. Creating a professional website

9. C. Engage in ongoing marketing efforts and networking

10. C. Exploring health insurance options through professional organizations

Chapter 23: Ethical Coding and Data Security

23.1. Ethics in Medical Coding

Ethics in medical coding is paramount, ensuring that all coding and billing practices are conducted with integrity, accuracy, and adherence to applicable laws and guidelines. Ethical coding practices protect patients' rights, ensure the correct use of healthcare resources, and maintain trust among healthcare providers, payers, and patients.

Principles of Ethical Medical Coding

1. Accuracy and Honesty:

- Coders must ensure that codes accurately reflect the patient's diagnosis and the services provided, without exaggeration or minimization to influence reimbursement.

2. Confidentiality and Privacy:

- Maintaining patient confidentiality is crucial. Coders must protect health information and adhere to regulations such as HIPAA (Health Insurance Portability and Accountability Act) in the

U.S., which sets standards for the protection of sensitive patient data.

3. Compliance with Laws and Regulations:

- Coders should stay informed about and comply with all relevant laws, regulations, and guidelines, including coding standards, payer policies, and federal and state laws.

4. Continuing Education:

- Ethical coding requires staying updated on the latest coding practices, guidelines, and regulatory changes. Continuous education is essential for maintaining coding integrity and professionalism.

5. Conflict of Interest Avoidance:

- Coders must avoid situations where personal interests could conflict with professional responsibilities. Transparency and disclosure of potential conflicts of interest are vital for ethical practice.

Challenges to Ethical Coding

- **Upcoding and Downcoding:** Deliberately coding for a higher level of service than provided (upcoding) or a lower level to avoid audits (downcoding) are unethical practices that can lead to significant legal and financial penalties.

- **Coder and Provider Pressures:** Coders may face pressure from employers or providers to code in a way that maximizes reimbursement, even if it doesn't accurately reflect the services provided.

- **Keeping Current with Coding Changes:** The constant evolution of coding guidelines and healthcare regulations can make it challenging for coders to stay informed and apply the latest standards accurately.

Strategies for Promoting Ethical Coding

1. Establish a Code of Ethics:

- Healthcare organizations should develop and enforce a clear code of ethics for coding practices, providing guidance on handling ethical dilemmas.

2. Regular Audits and Compliance Checks:

- Conducting regular coding audits can help identify and correct unethical coding practices, reinforcing the importance of accuracy and compliance.

3. Education and Training Programs:

- Implement ongoing education and training programs on ethical coding practices, new regulations, and the implications of unethical behavior.

4. Supportive Work Environment:

- Create a work environment that encourages ethical behavior, where coders feel supported in making ethical decisions and can report unethical practices without fear of retaliation.

5. Transparency with Patients:

- Ensure that billing statements to patients are accurate and transparent, allowing patients to understand the services billed and encouraging trust in the healthcare provider.

Conclusion

Ethical coding is foundational to the integrity of medical billing and the healthcare system as a whole. By adhering to principles of accuracy, confidentiality, and compliance, and by fostering an environment that supports ethical decision-making, medical coders play a crucial role in upholding the standards of healthcare provision and administration.

23.2. Data Security and Patient Confidentiality

In the realm of medical coding and healthcare, data security and patient confidentiality are paramount. The sensitive nature of patient health information mandates stringent measures to protect data from unauthorized access, breaches, and misuse.

Ensuring data security not only complies with legal requirements but also fosters trust between patients and healthcare providers.

Key Aspects of Data Security and Patient Confidentiality

1. Understanding HIPAA and Other Regulations:

- The Health Insurance Portability and Accountability Act (HIPAA) in the U.S., along with other global data protection regulations, sets standards for the protection of sensitive patient health information.

- Compliance involves adhering to privacy, security, and breach notification rules designed to safeguard patient data.

2. Implementing Strong Data Protection Measures:

- Healthcare organizations and medical coders must employ robust security measures, including encryption, secure data transmission protocols, and access controls, to protect health information stored electronically (ePHI) or in paper form.

3. Regular Training and Awareness Programs:

- Continuous education on data security practices and legal requirements for all staff involved in handling patient information is crucial.

- Training programs should cover topics such as secure handling of data, recognizing phishing attempts, and proper disposal of sensitive information.

4. Access Controls and Authentication:

- Implementing strict access controls ensures that only authorized personnel can access patient data. This includes using strong passwords, multi-factor authentication, and maintaining detailed access logs.

5. Incident Response and Breach Notification:

- Organizations must have an incident response plan in place to promptly address any data breaches or security incidents.

- In case of a breach, complying with breach notification laws involves informing affected patients and relevant authorities in a timely manner.

Challenges in Ensuring Data Security

- **Rapid Technological Advances:** Keeping pace with rapid changes in technology and evolving cyber threats can be challenging for healthcare organizations.

- **Insider Threats:** Unauthorized access or breaches by employees or contractors, whether intentional or accidental, pose significant risks to patient data security.

- **Third-Party Risks:** Sharing patient data with third parties, such as billing companies or cloud service providers, requires diligent oversight to ensure external compliance with data protection standards.

Strategies for Enhancing Data Security and Patient Confidentiality

1. Conducting Regular Risk Assessments:

- Identify potential vulnerabilities in your data protection measures and take proactive steps to mitigate risks.

2. Developing a Culture of Security:

- Foster a workplace culture where data security and patient confidentiality are prioritized and valued by all staff members.

3. Investing in Advanced Security Technologies:

- Leverage advanced security solutions, such as firewalls, anti-malware tools, and intrusion detection systems, to fortify defenses against cyber threats.

4. Establishing Clear Policies and Procedures:

- Develop and enforce clear policies regarding the handling, storage, and transmission of patient information, including protocols for mobile device usage and remote work.

5. Engaging with Cybersecurity Experts:

- Consider consulting with cybersecurity experts or hiring dedicated security professionals to ensure your data protection strategies are comprehensive and up-to-date.

Conclusion

Data security and patient confidentiality are critical components of medical coding and healthcare administration. By implementing rigorous security measures, complying with legal requirements, and fostering a culture of privacy and security, healthcare organizations can protect sensitive patient information and maintain the trust and confidence of patients and stakeholders.

23.3. Handling Sensitive Medical Information

Handling sensitive medical information with the utmost care and confidentiality is a fundamental responsibility of everyone in the healthcare industry, including medical coders. The sensitive nature of patient data requires stringent adherence to ethical standards, legal requirements, and best practices to protect patient privacy and ensure data security.

Principles for Handling Sensitive Medical Information

1. Understand and Comply with HIPAA Guidelines:

- Familiarize yourself with the Health Insurance Portability and Accountability Act (HIPAA) provisions, focusing on the Privacy Rule and Security Rule, which set standards for the protection and confidential handling of protected health information (PHI).

2. Ensure Minimum Necessary Use:

- Apply the "minimum necessary" standard when using or disclosing PHI, ensuring that only the minimum amount of information required to perform a task is accessed or shared.

3. Secure Storage and Transmission:

- Store patient information securely, using encrypted digital systems or locked cabinets for physical records. Ensure secure transmission of PHI, employing encryption for electronic transfers and cautious handling of physical documents.

4. Regular Training and Awareness:

- Participate in regular training sessions on data protection laws, organizational policies on privacy, and best practices for handling sensitive information. Staying informed about potential security threats and preventive measures is crucial.

Common Challenges in Handling Sensitive Medical Information

1. Cybersecurity Threats:

- Cyberattacks, such as phishing, malware, and ransomware, pose significant risks to the security of patient data.

- **Solution:** Implement comprehensive cybersecurity measures and conduct regular security awareness training for all staff.

2. Insider Threats:

- Unauthorized access or disclosure by employees, either unintentionally or maliciously, can compromise patient privacy.

- **Solution:** Enforce strict access controls, conduct background checks, and promote a culture of accountability and privacy.

3. Third-Party Data Sharing:

- Sharing information with third parties, including billing services and business associates, requires careful oversight to ensure they comply with privacy standards.

- **Solution:** Establish Business Associate Agreements (BAAs) and conduct regular audits of third-party vendors.

Best Practices for Handling Sensitive Medical Information

1. Access Controls and Authentication:

- Implement strong password policies, multi-factor authentication, and role-based access controls to limit access to PHI.

2. Data Encryption:

- Use encryption for storing and transmitting patient information to protect against unauthorized access.

3. Regular Audits and Monitoring:

- Conduct periodic audits of information access and usage to detect any unauthorized or inappropriate activity.

4. Clear Policies and Employee Training:

- Develop clear policies for handling PHI and provide ongoing employee training to reinforce these policies and procedures.

5. Incident Response Planning:

- Have an incident response plan in place to quickly address any breaches or security incidents, minimizing potential harm.

Conclusion

The handling of sensitive medical information is a critical aspect of healthcare that demands diligence, adherence to ethical and legal standards, and proactive measures to ensure data security. By implementing robust policies, investing in employee training, and utilizing technology wisely, healthcare professionals, including medical coders, can safeguard patient confidentiality and maintain the trust essential to healthcare delivery.

23.4. Legal Implications in Medical Coding

Medical coding not only requires a thorough understanding of healthcare terminology and coding systems but also an awareness of the legal implications associated with the practice. Legal issues in medical coding can arise from inaccuracies, non-compliance with regulations, and unethical coding practices, leading to significant consequences for healthcare providers and coding professionals.

Key Legal Implications in Medical Coding

1. Fraud and Abuse:

- **Overview:** Fraud involves intentionally submitting false claims or making misrepresentations to obtain payment, while abuse refers to practices that are not necessarily fraudulent but are inconsistent with sound fiscal or medical practices.

- **Consequences:** Penalties can include fines, exclusion from federal healthcare programs (e.g., Medicare and Medicaid), and even criminal charges.

2. Compliance with HIPAA:

- **Overview:** The Health Insurance Portability and Accountability Act (HIPAA) sets standards for the protection of patient health information. Non-compliance can occur if there's a failure to adequately protect patient data or if there's unauthorized access or disclosure.

- **Consequences:** Violations can lead to civil and criminal penalties, including fines and, in severe cases, imprisonment.

3. Accurate and Ethical Coding:

- **Overview:** Accurate coding is critical for proper billing and reimbursement. Upcoding, downcoding, and unbundling are examples of unethical coding practices that can lead to legal issues.

- **Consequences:** Such practices can result in claim denials, repayments, fines, and legal action for fraud.

4. False Claims Act (FCA):

- **Overview:** The FCA is a federal law that imposes liability on individuals and companies who defraud governmental programs. In the context of medical coding, this includes submitting claims for services not provided or coding services at a higher rate than provided.

- **Consequences:** Penalties can include treble damages (three times the amount of damages the government sustains) and penalties for each false claim.

Strategies for Avoiding Legal Issues in Medical Coding

1. Comprehensive Training and Education:

- Ensure coders and healthcare providers receive ongoing training on coding standards, legal requirements, and ethical practices.

2. Implementing Robust Compliance Programs:

- Develop and enforce a compliance program that includes regular audits, monitoring, and mechanisms for reporting and addressing compliance issues.

3. Use of Coding Audits:

- Conduct regular internal or external coding audits to identify and rectify inaccuracies before they result in legal issues.

4. Maintaining Transparency and Documentation:

- Keep detailed documentation of coding decisions and communications with healthcare providers to justify coding choices and facilitate audits.

5. Encouraging a Culture of Ethics and Compliance:

- Foster an organizational culture that emphasizes ethical behavior, compliance with laws and regulations, and the importance of accurate coding.

Conclusion

The legal implications in medical coding highlight the importance of accuracy, ethical practices, and compliance with regulations. By understanding the potential legal consequences and implementing strategies to mitigate risks, healthcare organizations and coding professionals can protect themselves from legal challenges and contribute to the integrity and sustainability of healthcare delivery.

23.5. Exercise: 10 MCQs with Answers at the End

Test your understanding of ethical coding, data security, handling sensitive medical information, and legal implications in medical coding. Answers are provided at the end for self-assessment.

Questions

1. What act sets standards for the protection of sensitive patient health information in the U.S.?

A. Affordable Care Act (ACA)

B. Health Insurance Portability and Accountability Act (HIPAA)

C. False Claims Act (FCA)

D. American Medical Association (AMA)

2. Deliberately coding for a higher level of service than was provided is known as:

A. Encryption

B. Upcoding

C. Data Mining

D. Compliance

3. Which of the following is NOT a principle of ethical medical coding?

A. Minimum necessary use

B. Regularly changing coding guidelines to fit needs

C. Confidentiality and privacy

D. Accuracy and honesty

4. Implementing strong passwords and multi-factor authentication are strategies for:

A. Avoiding audits

B. Ensuring data security

C. Marketing a coding business

D. Handling legal disputes

5. Regular training on data protection laws and best practices is essential for:

A. Only new employees

B. Healthcare providers but not coders

C. Everyone involved in handling patient information

D. External consultants only

6. Penalties for violating the Health Insurance Portability and Accountability Act (HIPAA) can include:

A. Fines only

B. Criminal charges only

C. Both fines and criminal charges

D. No consequences

7. The "minimum necessary" standard refers to:

A. Using the least amount of effort in coding

B. Using or disclosing only the minimum amount of patient information necessary

C. Minimum compliance with legal standards

D. The least amount of data encryption required

8. A compliance program for a medical coding department should NOT include:

A. Mechanisms for reporting compliance issues

B. Regular audits and monitoring

C. Incentives for upcoding to increase revenue

D. Comprehensive training and education

9. Which law imposes liability on individuals and companies who defraud governmental programs?

A. Health Information Technology for Economic and Clinical Health Act (HITECH)

B. False Claims Act (FCA)

C. Patient Protection and Affordable Care Act (ACA)

D. Health Maintenance Organization Act (HMO)

10. Ethical coding practices protect:

A. Only the coding professional

B. Only the healthcare provider

C. Patient rights and ensure correct healthcare resource use

D. The interests of insurance companies

Answers

1. B. Health Insurance Portability and Accountability Act (HIPAA)

2. B. Upcoding

3. B. Regularly changing coding guidelines to fit needs

4. B. Ensuring data security

5. C. Everyone involved in handling patient information

6. C. Both fines and criminal charges

7. B. Using or disclosing only the minimum amount of patient information necessary

8. C. Incentives for upcoding to increase revenue

9. B. False Claims Act (FCA)

10. C. Patient rights and ensure correct healthcare resource use

Chapter 24: Navigating the Global Coding Landscape

24.1. International Coding Standards

The field of medical coding extends beyond the borders of any single country, necessitating international coding standards to ensure consistency, accuracy, and efficiency in the global healthcare system. These standards facilitate the sharing of health information across different healthcare systems, support public health and research, and streamline billing and reimbursement processes internationally.

Key International Coding Standards

1. International Classification of Diseases (ICD):

- **Overview:** Developed by the World Health Organization (WHO), the ICD is the international standard for classifying diseases and health conditions. It is used globally for morbidity and mortality statistics, disease reporting, and epidemiology. The ICD-10 is the version currently in use, with ICD-11 released for implementation in member states.

- **Application:** The ICD is used by healthcare providers and payers worldwide to classify diseases on health records, track epidemiological trends, and compile global health statistics.

2. Systematized Nomenclature of Medicine -- Clinical Terms (SNOMED CT):

- **Overview:** SNOMED CT is a comprehensive, multilingual clinical healthcare terminology that provides precise terms for clinical documentation and reporting. It covers diseases, clinical findings, procedures, and outcomes, facilitating detailed clinical data capture.

- **Application:** Used in electronic health records (EHRs), it enhances the exchange and analysis of health data, supporting clinical decision-making and research.

3. Current Procedural Terminology (CPT) International:

- **Overview:** While CPT, developed by the American Medical Association (AMA), is primarily used in the United States for coding medical procedures and services, its principles and structure influence procedural coding standards in other countries.

- **Application:** Some countries have developed their procedural coding systems inspired by CPT or use CPT directly for specific purposes, such as clinical trials or research.

Challenges in International Coding Standards

- **Interoperability:** Ensuring compatibility and seamless exchange of health information across different coding systems and EHR technologies.

- **Language and Cultural Differences:** Adapting coding standards to different languages and cultural contexts while maintaining consistency and accuracy.

- **Training and Implementation:** Providing adequate training and resources for healthcare professionals worldwide to implement and adhere to international coding standards.

- **Data Privacy and Security:** Balancing the need for data sharing and analysis with the protection of patient privacy and adherence to varying national data protection laws.

Strategies for Navigating International Coding Standards

1. Global Collaboration and Harmonization:

- Engage in international efforts to harmonize coding standards and practices, such as WHO's initiatives for ICD implementation and the International Health Terminology Standards Development Organisation (IHTSDO) for SNOMED CT.

2. Continuous Education and Training:

- Provide ongoing education for medical coders and healthcare professionals on international coding standards, including updates and best practices for implementation.

3. Technology and Interoperability Solutions:

- Invest in EHR and coding software that supports multiple coding standards and offers interoperability solutions for the exchange of health information across borders.

4. Adaptation to Local Contexts:

- Customize international coding standards to fit local healthcare practices, language, and legal requirements, ensuring relevance and applicability.

Conclusion

International coding standards play a crucial role in global health information management, facilitating the accurate and consistent classification of health data worldwide. Navigating the global coding landscape requires a commitment to collaboration, education, and the use of technology to overcome challenges and harness the full potential of these standards for improving healthcare delivery and outcomes on a global scale.

24.2. Coding in Diverse Healthcare Systems

Navigating medical coding within diverse healthcare systems around the world presents unique challenges and opportunities. Different countries have their own healthcare policies, systems, and coding standards, which can significantly impact how medical coding is implemented and managed. Understanding these variances is crucial for global health information management and for professionals working in or with international healthcare systems.

Challenges of Coding in Diverse Healthcare Systems

1. Variability in Healthcare Delivery and Financing:

- Healthcare systems vary globally in terms of structure, delivery, and financing, from publicly funded systems to private insurance-based models. These differences can affect coding practices, reimbursement processes, and the importance placed on certain types of coding.

2. Different Coding Standards and Requirements:

- While the International Classification of Diseases (ICD) is widely used, countries may adopt different versions or modify them to suit local needs. Additionally, some countries have developed their own coding systems for procedures and services, adding another layer of complexity.

3. Language and Terminology Differences:

- Translating medical records and applying coding standards across languages can introduce inaccuracies. Medical terminology may not have direct equivalents in all languages, requiring careful consideration and sometimes adaptation of coding systems.

4. Varied Levels of Technology Adoption:

- The extent to which electronic health records (EHRs) and computer-assisted coding (CAC) systems are implemented varies, influencing coding efficiency, accuracy, and data analysis capabilities.

Strategies for Effective Coding Across Healthcare Systems

1. Global Collaboration and Standardization Efforts:

- Participating in international efforts to harmonize coding standards and practices can help address discrepancies and promote consistency. Organizations such as the World Health Organization (WHO) and the International Health Terminology Standards Development Organisation (IHTSDO) play key roles in these efforts.

2. Education and Training:

- Providing coders with comprehensive training that covers both global coding standards and specific local adaptations ensures they are well-equipped to handle coding tasks accurately across different systems.

3. Leveraging Technology for Interoperability:

- Investing in advanced EHR and CAC systems that support multiple coding standards and languages can enhance interoperability and accuracy in coding, facilitating international data exchange and analysis.

4. Cultural and Linguistic Adaptation:

- Developing coding resources and tools that accommodate linguistic diversity and cultural differences in healthcare practices can improve coding accuracy and relevance in diverse settings.

Conclusion

Coding in diverse healthcare systems requires an understanding of the unique challenges and opportunities presented by international variations in healthcare delivery, financing, and regulation. By adopting strategies for global collaboration, education, technological innovation, and cultural adaptation, the medical coding community can navigate these complexities, contributing to improved health information management and patient care worldwide.

24.3. Cross-Country Coding Challenges

Navigating the landscape of medical coding across different countries presents a unique set of challenges. These challenges stem from variations in healthcare policies, coding standards, and practices, as well as differences in language and legal requirements. Understanding these challenges is crucial for global health information management, especially for organizations operating in multiple countries or for professionals involved in international coding projects.

Key Cross-Country Coding Challenges

1. Variation in Coding Standards and Practices:

- Different countries may use various versions of the International Classification of Diseases (ICD) or have their own national coding systems, leading to discrepancies in how medical conditions and procedures are coded.

- **Strategy:** Engage in continuous education and training on international coding standards and the specific requirements of each country you work with.

2. Healthcare Policy and Reimbursement Models:

- The approach to healthcare financing varies significantly across countries, from public health systems to insurance-based models, impacting coding priorities and reimbursement processes.

- **Strategy:** Develop a thorough understanding of the healthcare systems in the countries you operate, focusing on how coding influences reimbursement and policy compliance.

3. Legal and Regulatory Compliance:

- Each country has its own legal framework and regulations governing patient data privacy, security, and medical billing, posing a challenge for maintaining compliance across borders.

- **Strategy:** Implement robust compliance programs that are adaptable to different regulatory environments, ensuring patient data is handled securely and legally.

4. Language Barriers and Cultural Differences:

- Medical terminology and patient records may need to be translated or adapted for different languages, increasing the risk of inaccuracies. Cultural differences can also influence medical practices and documentation.

- **Strategy:** Utilize professional translation services and culturally sensitive coding practices to ensure accuracy and appropriateness in coding across languages and cultures.

5. Technology and Infrastructure Disparities:

- The level of technological advancement and the adoption of electronic health records (EHRs) and computer-assisted coding (CAC) systems vary, affecting coding efficiency and data quality.

- **Strategy:** Leverage cloud-based EHR and coding solutions that offer flexibility and scalability across different technological environments.

Overcoming Cross-Country Coding Challenges

- **International Collaboration:** Participate in global health information management initiatives and forums to share knowledge, best practices, and collaborate on overcoming common coding challenges.

- **Customization and Localization:** Tailor coding practices and software solutions to meet the specific needs of each country, considering local languages, legal requirements, and healthcare practices.

- **Advanced Training for Coders:** Provide specialized training for medical coders that covers not only international coding standards like ICD but also country-specific coding guidelines and cultural considerations.

- **Use of Interoperable Systems:** Invest in health information systems that support interoperability and can accommodate different coding standards and languages, facilitating accurate and efficient coding across countries.

Conclusion

Cross-country coding challenges require a strategic approach that combines education, technology, and international collaboration. By addressing these challenges proactively, healthcare organizations and coding professionals can ensure accurate, efficient, and compliant coding practices that support global health information management and patient care.

24.4. International Career Opportunities in Coding

The globalization of healthcare and advancements in technology have expanded career opportunities for medical coders beyond their home countries. With a growing demand for accurate and standardized health information management across the globe, skilled coders now have various avenues to explore international careers. These opportunities not only offer professional growth but also the chance to contribute to global health initiatives.

Key Areas for International Career Opportunities

1. Telecommuting for International Healthcare Providers:

- Many healthcare providers and medical coding companies now offer remote coding positions, allowing coders to work for organizations located in different countries without the need to relocate.

2. Global Health Organizations:

- Organizations such as the World Health Organization (WHO) and non-governmental organizations (NGOs) involved in global health initiatives may require coding expertise for research, data analysis, and health information management projects.

3. Health Information Technology Companies:

- With the increasing adoption of electronic health records (EHRs) and health information systems worldwide, technology companies seek medical coders to contribute to software development, implementation, and training projects across different countries.

4. Medical Tourism:

- The growing industry of medical tourism, where patients travel internationally for medical care, creates a demand for coders who can navigate multiple healthcare systems and coding standards.

5. Consulting and Education:

- Experienced coders can find opportunities in consulting, offering their expertise to healthcare facilities worldwide on coding practices, compliance, and optimization. Additionally, international training and education roles are available for coders to teach coding standards and practices.

Strategies for Pursuing International Opportunities

1. Gain International Coding Certifications:

- Obtaining certifications recognized internationally, such as those offered by the American Health Information Management Association (AHIMA) or the American Academy of Professional Coders (AAPC), can enhance your qualifications.

2. Develop Language Skills:

- Learning a second language relevant to the region you are interested in can be advantageous, especially for roles requiring interaction with local healthcare providers or patients.

3. Network Internationally:

- Participate in international coding forums, join global professional organizations, and attend international healthcare conferences to build connections and learn about opportunities.

4. Stay Informed About Global Health Trends:

- Understanding global health challenges, international healthcare policies, and trends in health information technology can make you more competitive for international roles.

5. Highlight Cross-Cultural Competence:

- In your resume and interviews, emphasize experiences or skills that demonstrate your ability to work effectively across different cultures and healthcare systems.

Challenges and Considerations

- **Legal and Regulatory Compliance:** Ensure you understand the legal and regulatory requirements for working internationally, including visa regulations and data protection laws.

- **Cultural Sensitivity:** Being aware of and sensitive to cultural differences is crucial when working in international settings or with diverse teams.

- **Time Zones:** Be prepared to navigate the challenges of working across time zones, which may require flexibility in your work schedule.

Conclusion

The demand for skilled medical coders in the global healthcare market presents numerous opportunities for professional growth and international experience. By acquiring relevant certifications, building language skills, and networking, coders can position themselves for successful careers that cross borders and contribute to improving healthcare delivery and outcomes worldwide.

24.5. Exercise: 10 MCQs with Answers at the End

Test your knowledge on navigating the global coding landscape, including international coding standards, coding in diverse healthcare systems, cross-country coding challenges, and international career opportunities in coding. Answers are provided at the end for self-assessment.

Questions

1. Which organization develops the ICD coding system?

   A. WHO

   B. AAPC

   C. AHIMA

   D. NHS

2. SNOMED CT is primarily used for:

   A. Billing and reimbursement

   B. Clinical documentation and reporting

   C. International travel health advisories

   D. Medical equipment classification

3. The "minimum necessary" standard is a principle of:

   A. Financial auditing

   B. Ethical coding

   C. Data security

   D. Healthcare marketing

4. A major challenge in international medical coding is:

   A. Standardization of medical equipment

B. Language and terminology differences

C. Universal healthcare coverage

D. Global drug formularies

5. Telecommuting for international healthcare providers is an example of:

A. A coding certification

B. A global health organization

C. An international career opportunity

D. A health information technology company

6. Which is NOT a recognized international coding certification?

A. CPC

B. CCS

C. RN

D. CIC

7. Effective strategies for navigating cross-country coding challenges include:

A. Limiting coding to domestic cases only

B. Ignoring updates to international coding standards

C. Global collaboration and standardization efforts

D. Reducing reliance on technology in coding

8. The False Claims Act is related to:

A. International travel regulations

B. Legal implications in medical coding

C. Global health organization operations

D. Language translation services

9. HIPAA compliance is crucial for:

A. Only coders within the United States

B. Coders working internationally with U.S. patient data

C. Only healthcare providers outside the U.S.

D. International hotel chains offering medical tourism

10. A strategy for pursuing international coding opportunities is:

A. Avoiding professional development

B. Focusing solely on local coding standards

C. Gaining international coding certifications

D. Networking only within one's own country

Answers

1. A. WHO

2. B. Clinical documentation and reporting

3. B. Ethical coding

4. B. Language and terminology differences

5. C. An international career opportunity

6. C. RN

7. C. Global collaboration and standardization efforts

8. B. Legal implications in medical coding

9. B. Coders working internationally with U.S. patient data

10. C. Gaining international coding certifications

Chapter 25: The Future of Medical Coding

25.1. Emerging Trends in Healthcare and Coding

The field of medical coding is continuously evolving, shaped by advancements in technology, changes in healthcare policies, and the growing complexity of healthcare delivery. Staying abreast of emerging trends is essential for coding professionals to remain effective and adapt to the changing landscape. Here's a look at some of the significant trends influencing the future of medical coding.

Integration of Artificial Intelligence and Machine Learning

- **Overview:** Artificial intelligence (AI) and machine learning (ML) are increasingly being integrated into coding processes to enhance accuracy, efficiency, and to automate routine tasks. AI algorithms can analyze clinical documentation to suggest appropriate codes, reducing the time and potential for human error.

- **Impact:** Coders will need to adapt to new workflows that incorporate AI and ML, focusing more on validating AI-generated codes and managing complex coding cases that require human expertise.

Adoption of Natural Language Processing (NLP)

- **Overview:** NLP technology is being used to interpret and extract relevant information from unstructured clinical documentation. This assists coders by highlighting key diagnostic and procedural details that inform accurate code assignment.

- **Impact:** The adoption of NLP will necessitate coders to become proficient in working with technology that pre-analyzes clinical notes, allowing them to focus on nuanced coding decisions and quality assurance.

Increased Focus on Data Analytics

- **Overview:** There is a growing emphasis on the use of healthcare data for analytics, quality improvement, and population health management. Medical coders play a crucial role in ensuring the data entered into healthcare databases is accurate and comprehensive.

- **Impact:** Coders may find roles expanding into data quality management, analytics, and reporting, requiring skills in data analysis and interpretation.

Telehealth and Remote Services Coding

- **Overview:** The expansion of telehealth services, accelerated by the COVID-19 pandemic, has introduced new coding categories and guidelines for remote healthcare delivery.

- **Impact:** Coders need to stay updated on telehealth coding guidelines and be adaptable to code a broader range of services delivered via digital platforms.

Value-Based Care and Coding for Outcomes

- **Overview:** The shift towards value-based care emphasizes outcomes and patient satisfaction over the volume of services provided. This shift affects coding practices, as coders must accurately capture data that reflects the quality and effectiveness of care.

- **Impact:** Coders will need to understand the nuances of coding for value-based care programs and ensure documentation supports quality reporting and reimbursement models based on patient outcomes.

Global Standardization and Interoperability

- **Overview:** Efforts to standardize coding practices and achieve interoperability among health information systems globally are gaining momentum. This facilitates the sharing of health information across borders and healthcare systems.

- **Impact:** Coders may increasingly work with international coding standards and need to be aware of global health data exchange protocols.

Conclusion

The future of medical coding is dynamic, with emerging trends highlighting the importance of technology, data analytics, and changing healthcare delivery models. As the field evolves, coders will need to embrace continuous learning and adaptability to navigate these changes successfully. Opportunities for coders to expand their roles and contribute to broader healthcare objectives are on the horizon, emphasizing the critical role of coding in the healthcare ecosystem.

25.2. The Evolving Role of Medical Coders

The landscape of medical coding is undergoing significant transformation, driven by advancements in technology, shifts in healthcare policies, and the growing emphasis on data-driven care. These changes are not only reshaping the tasks and responsibilities of medical coders but also expanding their roles within the healthcare industry.

From Coding to Data Management

- **Overview:** As automation and artificial intelligence (AI) begin to take on more of the routine coding tasks, coders are transitioning towards roles that emphasize data management, analysis, and quality assurance.

- **Impact:** Coders are increasingly becoming stewards of medical data, ensuring its accuracy, completeness, and integrity for billing, reporting, and analytics purposes.

Enhanced Focus on Data Quality and Analytics

- **Overview:** With the shift towards value-based care and the use of big data in healthcare, the focus on data quality has never been more critical. Coders are at the forefront of capturing clinical data that informs patient care, reimbursement, and health outcomes analysis.

- **Impact:** Coders need to develop skills in data analytics and understand the implications of coding on healthcare outcomes, quality reporting, and financial performance.

Increased Specialization

- **Overview:** The complexity of medical treatments and the nuances of coding rules are leading coders to specialize in specific areas of healthcare, such as oncology, cardiology, or outpatient services.

- **Impact:** Specialization allows coders to deepen their expertise in particular domains, enhancing their value to healthcare organizations and opening up opportunities for career advancement.

Role in Compliance and Audit Readiness

- **Overview:** Coders play a pivotal role in ensuring compliance with coding guidelines, payer policies, and regulatory requirements. Their expertise is essential for preparing for and responding to audits.

- **Impact:** Coders must stay abreast of the latest coding standards and regulations, often taking on roles that involve compliance monitoring, education, and internal auditing.

Engagement in Healthcare IT and EHR Optimization

- **Overview:** The integration of Electronic Health Records (EHRs) and other health IT systems into everyday healthcare practices has created a demand for coders who are proficient in these technologies.

- **Impact:** Coders are involved in EHR system optimization, ensuring that these systems support accurate and efficient coding, and contributing to the design and testing of health IT solutions.

Education and Training

- **Overview:** As the coding profession evolves, there is a growing need for coders to engage in continuous education and training, not only on coding standards but also on emerging healthcare trends and technologies.

- **Impact:** Coders may find opportunities as educators and trainers, sharing their knowledge with peers, healthcare providers, and coding students.

Conclusion

The evolving role of medical coders reflects the broader changes occurring within the healthcare industry. As their traditional tasks become more automated, coders are stepping into roles that require a broader skill set, including data management, compliance, health IT, and education. This evolution presents coders with new challenges but also opportunities for professional growth and greater involvement in the critical processes that drive healthcare quality and efficiency.

25.3. Innovations in Coding Practices

The medical coding field is experiencing significant transformations due to technological advancements and changing healthcare dynamics. These innovations aim to improve accuracy, efficiency, and the overall effectiveness of coding practices, thus impacting healthcare billing, compliance, and data analysis. Here's a look at some of the key innovations shaping the future of medical coding.

Artificial Intelligence (AI) and Machine Learning (ML) in Coding

- **Overview:** AI and ML technologies are increasingly being applied to automate the coding process, from extracting relevant information from electronic health records (EHRs) to suggesting accurate codes based on clinical documentation.

- **Impact:** These technologies reduce the time spent on manual coding, minimize errors, and allow coders to focus on more complex cases that require human expertise.

Natural Language Processing (NLP) for Documentation Review

- **Overview:** NLP technology interprets free-text clinical documentation, identifying key terms and phrases related to diagnoses and procedures that inform coding decisions.

- **Impact:** NLP facilitates a more efficient review of clinical documentation, enhancing the accuracy of code assignment and reducing the need for extensive manual review.

Blockchain for Data Integrity and Security

- **Overview:** Blockchain technology offers a secure, decentralized way to manage health records and coding information, ensuring data integrity and traceability.

- **Impact:** Implementing blockchain can significantly improve the security of coding data, reduce fraud, and enhance the reliability of health information exchange between entities.

Telehealth Coding and Reimbursement

- **Overview:** The rise of telehealth services, especially during the COVID-19 pandemic, has led to the development of specific coding guidelines and reimbursement policies for remote healthcare services.

- **Impact:** Coders must stay informed about telehealth coding regulations and ensure accurate coding for these services, addressing the unique challenges of documenting and billing for virtual care.

Predictive Analytics for Coding and Compliance

- **Overview:** Predictive analytics uses historical data to identify trends and predict future outcomes related to coding practices, billing patterns, and potential compliance issues.

- **Impact:** By leveraging predictive analytics, healthcare organizations can proactively address coding and billing issues, optimize revenue cycle management, and improve compliance strategies.

Interoperability and Standardized Coding

- **Overview:** Efforts towards interoperability aim to standardize coding practices across different healthcare systems and EHR platforms, facilitating seamless data exchange and communication.

- **Impact:** Standardization and interoperability improve the consistency and accuracy of coding across healthcare settings, enhancing patient care coordination and data analysis for public health.

Continuous Education and Training Platforms

- **Overview:** Online platforms and digital resources are increasingly available for coders to stay updated on coding guidelines, healthcare regulations, and innovations in coding technology.

- **Impact:** Continuous access to education and training ensures that coders can adapt to new technologies and changes in the coding landscape, maintaining their expertise and contributing to the quality of healthcare documentation and billing.

Conclusion

Innovations in medical coding practices are set to redefine the role of coders, making coding more accurate, efficient, and secure. As these technologies continue to evolve, coders will need to embrace continuous learning and adaptability to navigate the future of coding successfully. The integration of these innovations presents an opportunity to enhance the value coders bring to healthcare organizations, ultimately impacting patient care and the healthcare industry's financial health.

25.4. Preparing for the Future in Medical Coding

As the healthcare industry evolves with technological advancements and regulatory changes, medical coders must proactively prepare for the future. Embracing new technologies, acquiring advanced skills, and staying informed about industry trends are essential steps for coders to remain relevant and contribute effectively to the healthcare sector. Here's how medical coders can prepare for the future.

Embrace Technological Innovations

- **Stay Informed:** Keep abreast of emerging technologies in healthcare coding, such as AI, ML, and NLP, and understand how they impact coding processes.

- **Skill Development:** Pursue training in health information technology, including EHR systems and coding software, to enhance your technological proficiency.

Continuous Education and Certification

- **Coding Standards and Regulations:** Regularly update your knowledge of coding guidelines, including ICD, CPT, and HCPCS updates, and understand the implications of healthcare regulations such as HIPAA.

- **Advanced Certifications:** Consider obtaining advanced coding certifications or specializations in areas like risk adjustment coding, compliance, or data analytics to broaden your expertise.

Develop Analytical and Soft Skills

- **Data Analytics:** As coding increasingly contributes to data-driven healthcare decisions, coders should develop skills in data analysis and interpretation.

- **Communication and Collaboration:** Enhance your communication and collaboration skills to work effectively with healthcare providers, IT professionals, and administrative staff.

Participate in Professional Networks

- **Networking:** Engage with professional coding associations, online forums, and social media groups dedicated to medical coding to exchange knowledge and stay connected with industry developments.

- **Conferences and Workshops:** Attend coding conferences, seminars, and workshops to learn from experts, discover innovations, and network with peers.

Adapt to New Coding Practices

- **Telehealth and Remote Services:** Familiarize yourself with coding for telehealth services, understanding the specific guidelines and challenges associated with remote healthcare delivery.

- **Value-Based Care:** Learn about coding for value-based care models, focusing on how coding accuracy affects quality measures, patient outcomes, and reimbursement.

Understand Global Healthcare Trends

- **International Standards:** For those working in or with international healthcare settings, understanding global coding standards and practices is crucial.

- **Cross-Cultural Competence:** Develop cultural competence to effectively navigate coding and healthcare practices in diverse international contexts.

Focus on Quality and Compliance

- **Quality Assurance:** Engage in or contribute to quality assurance processes within your organization, ensuring coding accuracy and compliance.

- **Ethical Practices:** Uphold ethical coding practices, understanding the legal and financial implications of coding decisions.

Conclusion

Preparing for the future in medical coding requires a multifaceted approach that encompasses embracing technology, pursuing continuous education, developing a broad skill set, and staying engaged with the professional community. By taking proactive steps to adapt to changes and challenges in the field, medical coders can ensure their roles remain vital and impactful within the evolving landscape of healthcare.

25.5. Exercise: 10 MCQs with Answers at the End

Test your understanding of the future of medical coding, including emerging trends, the evolving role of medical coders, innovations in coding practices, and strategies for preparing for future changes in the field. Answers are provided at the end for self-assessment.

Questions

1. Which technology is increasingly being integrated into medical coding to enhance accuracy and efficiency?

   A. Artificial Intelligence (AI)

   B. Virtual Reality (VR)

   C. Blockchain

   D. Augmented Reality (AR)

2. Natural Language Processing (NLP) technology is primarily used for:

   A. Interpreting and extracting relevant information from clinical documentation.

   B. Creating virtual coding environments.

   C. Securing patient data through encryption.

   D. Facilitating remote patient consultations.

3. The shift towards which care model emphasizes coding for outcomes and patient satisfaction?

   A. Fee-for-service

   B. Value-based care

   C. Capitation

   D. Direct primary care

4. Continuous education for medical coders is essential for staying updated on:

A. Only ICD-10 updates.

B. New healthcare regulations and coding guidelines.

C. Basic computer skills.

D. Historical medical practices.

5. Which of the following skills is increasingly important for medical coders due to the use of healthcare data for analytics?

A. Data analysis

B. Typing speed

C. Graphic design

D. Web development

6. Specialization in areas like oncology or cardiology coding can:

A. Limit a coder's job opportunities.

B. Decrease a coder's market value.

C. Enhance a coder's expertise and marketability.

D. Make it harder to stay updated on coding changes.

7. Participating in professional networks and attending coding conferences can help coders:

   A. Avoid learning about new coding technologies.

   B. Stay isolated from industry developments.

   C. Exchange knowledge and stay connected with industry developments.

   D. Focus solely on local coding standards.

8. Advanced certifications in medical coding:

   A. Are no longer necessary due to AI.

   B. Can broaden a coder's expertise and career opportunities.

   C. Only apply to coding in the United States.

   D. Decrease the need for continuous education.

9. Preparing for the future in medical coding includes developing skills in:

   A. Only traditional coding practices.

   B. Data analysis and health information technology.

   C. Manual record-keeping.

   D. Avoiding use of electronic health records (EHRs).

10. Blockchain technology in medical coding can improve:

    A. Only the speed of coding.

    B. Data integrity and security.

    C. The physical health of coders.

    D. The use of VR in coding.

Answers

1. A. Artificial Intelligence (AI)

2. A. Interpreting and extracting relevant information from clinical documentation.

3. B. Value-based care

4. B. New healthcare regulations and coding guidelines.

5. A. Data analysis

6. C. Enhance a coder's expertise and marketability.

7. C. Exchange knowledge and stay connected with industry developments.

8. B. Can broaden a coder's expertise and career opportunities.

9. B. Data analysis and health information technology.

10. B. Data integrity and security.

Conclusion

As we conclude our exploration of the multifaceted world of medical coding, it's clear that this field is not only foundational to the healthcare industry but is also rapidly evolving. From the intricacies of coding standards and practices to the impact of emerging technologies like AI and blockchain, medical coding stands at the intersection of healthcare, technology, and data management.

The future of medical coding promises further integration of technological innovations, which will streamline processes, enhance accuracy, and open new avenues for coders to contribute to healthcare beyond traditional coding tasks. As the role of medical coders expands into areas such as data analysis, compliance, and health information technology, continuous education and adaptability will be key to navigating these changes successfully.

Moreover, the global coding landscape highlights the importance of standardization and interoperability in fostering a more connected and efficient global healthcare system. The challenges and opportunities presented by international coding practices underscore the need for coders to possess a broad skill set that encompasses technical knowledge, cultural competence, and an understanding of global health trends.

In preparing for the future, medical coders are encouraged to embrace continuous learning, engage with professional communities, and explore specialization areas that align with emerging healthcare priorities. By doing so, coders can ensure their skills remain relevant and that they are well-positioned to take advantage of new career opportunities that arise as the field evolves.

As we look ahead, the importance of ethical coding practices, data security, and patient confidentiality remains paramount. Coders play a critical role in upholding these standards, ensuring that patient data is handled with the utmost care and that coding practices reflect the integrity of the healthcare profession.

In summary, the future of medical coding is bright, with ample opportunities for professional growth and innovation. By staying informed about industry developments, embracing new technologies, and prioritizing ethical practices, medical coders can continue to make significant contributions to the healthcare industry and patient care.

The best way to thank an author is to write a review.